Massage

FOR HEALTH, RELAXATION AND VITALITY

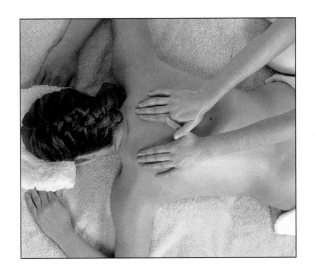

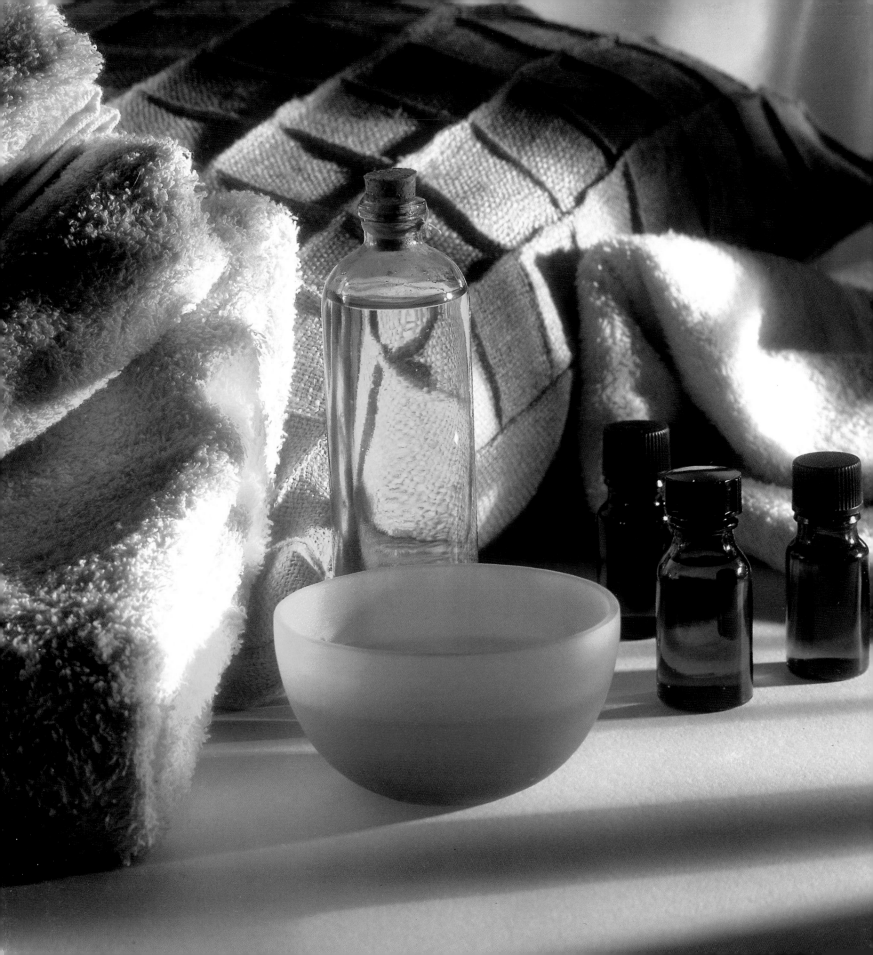

Massage

FOR HEALTH, RELAXATION AND VITALITY

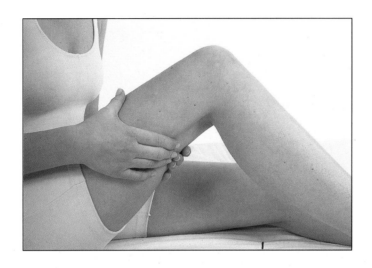

SARAH PORTER

LORENZ BOOKS

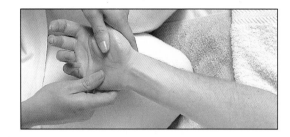

First published in 1998 by Lorenz Books

LORENZ BOOKS are available for bulk purchase, for sales promotion and
for premium use. For details, write or call the sales director, Lorenz Books,
27 West 20th Street, New York, NY 10011; (800) 354-9657

Lorenz Books is an imprint of
Anness Publishing Inc.

ISBN 1 85967 855 6

Publisher: Joanna Lorenz
Editor: Sarah Ainley
Copy Editor: Beverley Jollands
Designer: Bobbie Colgate Stone
Photographers: Sue Atkinson and Don Last

ACKNOWLEDGMENTS
The publishers would like to thank the following for their valuable contributions to this book:
Mark Evans, Kay Kiernan, Nitya Lacroix, Carole McGilvery, Lisa Myhill, Sharon Seager,
Jimi Reed, Karin Weisensel and Janice Welch

PICTURE CREDITS
Visual Arts Library: pp7, 8 and 9

PUBLISHER'S NOTE
The reader should not regard the recommendations, ideas and techniques
expressed and described in this book as substitutes for the advice of a qualified
practitioner or other qualified professional. Any use to which recommendations,
ideas and techniques are put is at the reader's sole discretion.

Printed in Hong Kong/China

1 3 5 7 9 10 8 6 4 2

CONTENTS

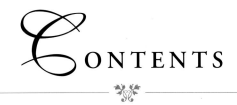

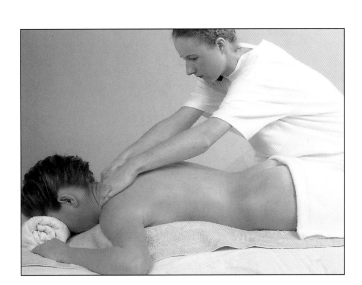

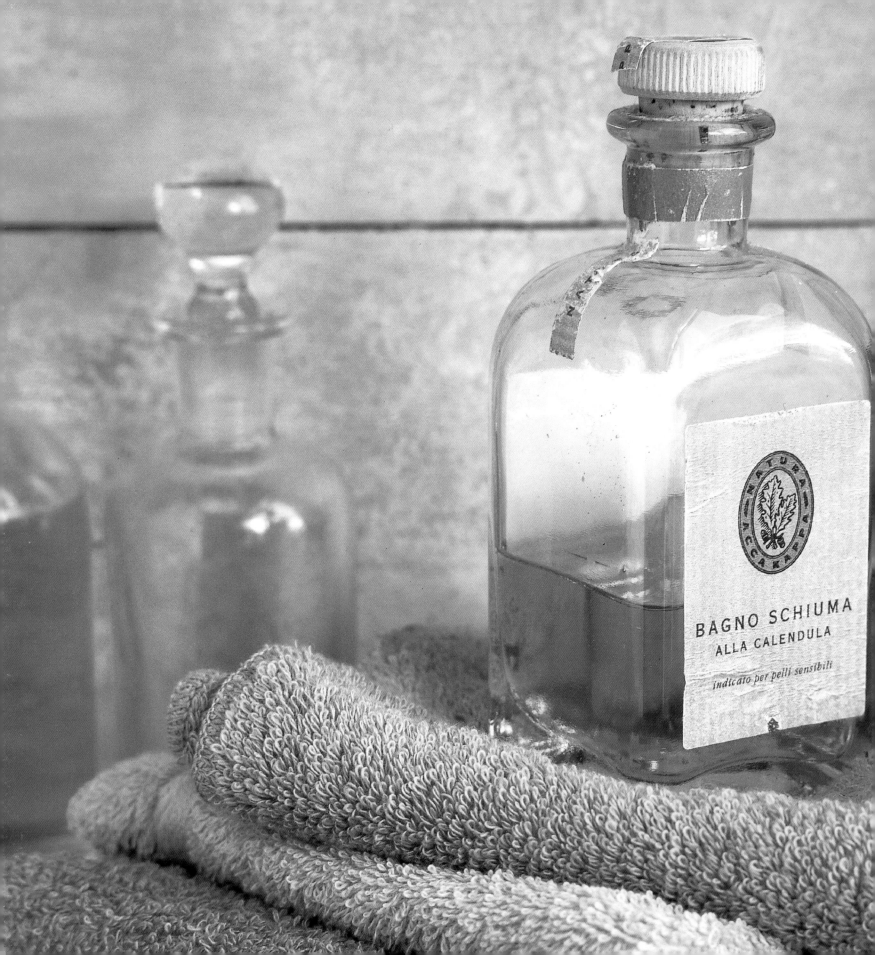

$\mathcal{I}$NTRODUCTION

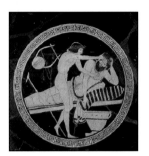

The sense of touch is a powerful and highly sensitive form of communication. It is a natural reaction to reach out and touch, whether to feel the shape or texture of an object, or to respond to – perhaps to comfort – another person. A mother cuddles her baby, everyone strokes the family pets, loving partners caress, and if you accidentally bump into something, you instinctively rub the sore spot better.

To touch someone can mean different things in different cultures. There are many social restraints which inhibit touching in public. In western society, a formal handshake, a nod of the head or a peck on each cheek are all recognized forms of greeting, and can be carried out without any show of real emotion. This rather formal approach to physical contact is contrary to our most basic instincts and needs. Fortunately, we are now rediscovering the healing power of massage and other touch therapies, which have been understood in other cultures for thousands of years.

Massage is beneficial to the whole physiological system: it stimulates and warms the tissues, improves blood flow and the elimination of toxins, and soothes the nervous system by inducing a state of deep relaxation. It provides a safe and neutral situation in which to receive the loving touch that is so important for our emotional health and self-esteem.

THE ART OF MASSAGE

Massage can fairly claim to be the oldest form of healing in existence. The use of touch to relieve aching muscles, to give comfort or to express love is as old as humankind, and is something humans share with animals as an instinctive way of bonding and sharing. As a stress-reliever it is probably without equal, and every culture throughout history has used massage in some form: every language, ancient or modern, has a word for massage.

AN ANCIENT TRADITION

Written records mentioning massage date back some 5000 years. *The Yellow Emperor's Classic of Internal Medicine* advocated stroking the limbs to "protect against colds, keep the organs supple and prevent minor ailments". Ancient Sanskrit texts advocate the benefits of massage, and in India, the Ayurvedic scriptures, which are nearly 4000 years old, also recommend rubbing and shampooing the body to keep it healthy and to promote healing. The tradition of using massage has remained unbroken in India since that time: most mothers are taught to massage their newborn babies, and when they grow up the children are taught to massage their parents.

MASSAGE IN THE CLASSICAL WORLD

In ancient Greece the practice of rubbing up the limbs, or *anatripsis*, was highly recommended for treating fatigue, sports or battle injuries and illness. Hippocrates, the so-called "father" of medicine, writing in the fifth century BC, stated that the physician must be "experienced in many things but assuredly rubbing". He suggested that the way to health was to have a scented bath and an oiled massage every day. Greek medical centres, or

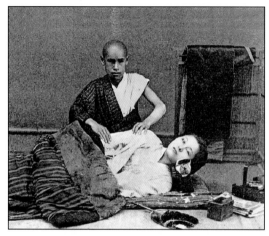

The Chinese have long believed in the therapeutic properties inherent in regular massage. Gentle manipulation of the limbs was said to have an improving effect on the circulation.

gymnasia, as they were known, nearly always included massage schools within them.

The Romans were equally enthusiastic about the benefits of massage, incorporating it into a daily routine in their spas alongside hot and cold baths; Julius Caesar had regular massages in an attempt to cure his epilepsy. The renowned Roman physician, Galen, wrote 16 manuals on the subject of massage, and introduced a variety of techniques and strokes that are still commonly used in massage today.

Massage continued to be popular and respected in Europe after the end of Roman rule, although the elaborate Roman baths and massage facilities soon fell into disrepair. But with the rise of Christianity, the needs of the body came to be seen as self-indulgent and sinful, and massage was neglected.

THE FOUNDATIONS OF MODERN MASSAGE

From the time of the Renaissance, when classical medicine and philosophy were once again in favour, massage was revived and respected once more. In 14th-century France, the physician Guy de Chauliac wrote a classic textbook in which he promoted hands-on techniques of manipulation as being highly complementary to surgical science.

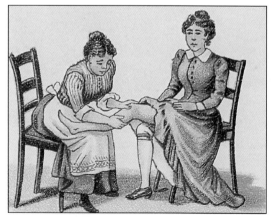

Massage strokes were often recommended as cures for common ailments in the late 19th century.

With the spread of the Ottoman Empire came Turkish-style bath and massage treatments. As the benefits of regular body work were recognized, massage became a firmly established part of beauty rituals for the wealthy.

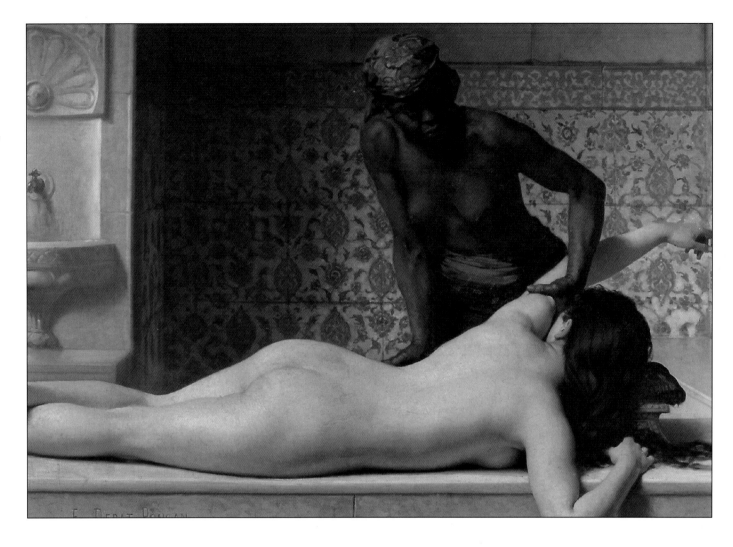

The foundations of modern massage and physiotherapy are based on a system devised by the Swede, Per Henrik Ling (1776–1839). Ling studied the human body in activity and at rest, and developed a system of medical gymnastics, exercises and massage, based upon ancient techniques learned while travelling through China. His research led to a royal appointment and the formation of an institute of massage. Ling's classification of strokes forms the basis of modern western massage.

HOLISTIC MASSAGE

Holistic massage, as described in this book, is the most popular of recent developments in massage. Recognizing the mind, body and spirit connection, holistic therapy looks at releasing trapped emotional issues and creating overall health and balance, rather than simply easing tired muscles and aching limbs.

The return to the premise that the caring touch is itself a powerful agent makes holistic massage suitable for a varied list of treatments. The massage uses the basic strokes of Swedish massage but works more gently, with the emphasis on relaxing the client psychologically and emotionally, as well as physically. The focus on relaxation applies to the practitioner as well, so that the experience has a calm and meditative quality for both people. The strokes remain important to the treatment, but it is the caring and loving quality of the touch that is fundamental to the holistic principle.

THE EFFECTS OF MASSAGE

When applied with skill and care, massage can evoke many beneficial changes within the body, mind and spirit. While the strokes ease pain and tension from stiff and aching muscles, boost a sluggish circulation or eliminate toxins, the nurturing touch of the hands soothes away mental stress and restores emotional equilibrium.

THE IMPORTANCE OF TOUCH

Massage provides a safe and neutral situation in which to receive the caring touch, which is so important for emotional health and self-esteem. Touch is fundamental to the development of a healthy human being, but the need to be touched does not stop with the end of childhood. Unfortunately, in many societies, physical contact between adults is strictly limited to intimate relationships.

The loving touch of massage unlocks not only the physical tensions trapped in muscles, but also acknowledges, with complete acceptance, the essence of the person within. While the massage itself is active, the underlying quality of the touch is one of stillness and calm, at one with the person receiving it. This is why massage is so beneficial; it helps you to feel safe enough to relax and unwind from the deepest parts of your mind.

REDUCING STRESS

Massage allows time for the replenishment of innate resources of vital energy. This is particularly relevant in the modern world when stress is known to be the root cause of many serious physical and mental conditions. Stress is a natural factor of life, but if it is not discharged appropriately, or is prolonged unduly, it robs the body of health and energy.

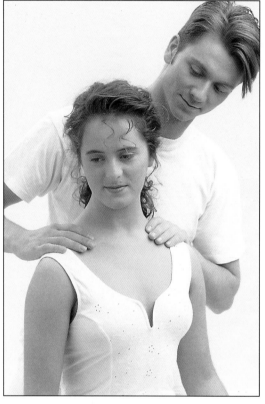

The power of touch easily transcends more formal means of communication as a pathway to deeper relaxation, increased vitality and greater self-awareness, to the benefit of both body and soul.

Stress can also lower the natural defences of the immune system. If you are constantly exposed to the adverse effects of stress, it can lead to anxiety, depression, lethargy, insomnia and panic attacks. Massage is increasingly recognized as a successful treatment for the symptoms arising from stress.

PHYSIOLOGICAL BENEFITS

Massage can both stimulate and relax the body. The skin, blood and lymphatic systems are all stimulated, boosting circulation, aiding cellular renewal and removing toxic waste. As tense muscles relax, stiff joints loosen and nerves are soothed, and an all-over feeling of relaxation and well-being is induced.

The nervous system

The nervous system is a highly complex network which relays messages from the brain to the rest of the body. The part of the nervous system that regulates many physiological functions leaves the brain at the base of the skull and runs down the spinal cord, protected by the spine's bony vertebrae. Depending on the depth of the movements used, the nerve endings can be stimulated or soothed in massage.

The skin

With massage comes an increase in blood circulation. This helps the exfoliation of superficial dead skin cells, tones the skin and encourages its renewal process. Massage helps to maintain the collagen fibres, which give skin its elasticity and strength and keep wrinkles at bay. The activity of the sweat and sebaceous glands, which lubricate and moisturize the skin, is regulated.

Muscles

With the increase in blood flow, the blood's vital nutrients circulate more efficiently. Massage is popular with sportspeople because it can improve muscle tone, restore mobility and ensure the elimination of waste products after exercise. Regular massage helps strains and sprains to heal more rapidly, and relaxes calf cramps and stiff muscles. Massage before an exercise session will help loosen and warm up the muscles; afterwards it will ease sore and aching limbs.

Circulation and lymphatic systems

By dilating the blood vessels, massage helps to increase the blood circulation, vital for the healthy functioning of the whole body.

At the same time, improved blood circulation helps accelerate the lymphatic system, which absorbs and eliminates waste products. Massage is an important way of speeding up the flow of lymph, thus providing the body with a strong immune system to fight against infections and disease.

The digestive system

Massage mobilizes the digestive system, helping problems such as constipation and flatulence. The digestive system is quick to respond to stress, and the reduction in tension that comes with regular massage has a regulating effect on the digestion.

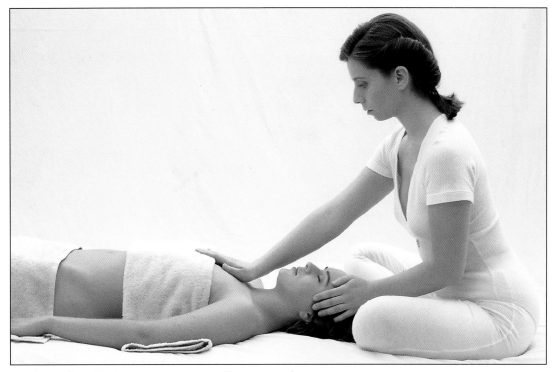

A calm and meditative environment contributes greatly to the therapeutic effect of a massage. Let go of any mental tensions before you begin as these can compromise the mood you are creating.

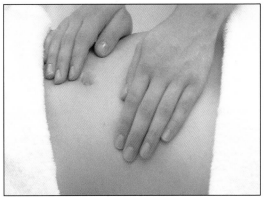

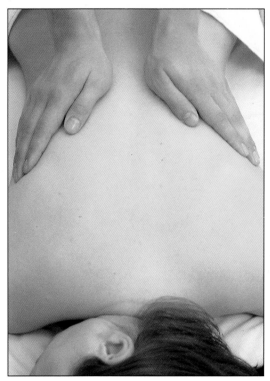

Placing your hands on the body of someone else can be one of the most direct ways to make contact with their inner being and help them to relax.

Massage allows an opportunity to connect with the energy of another person, and this in turn will help to increase your own sensitivity.

MASSAGE OILS

Throughout the world, people giving massage use locally available oils, usually vegetable oils, to help the hands flow and glide over the skin. Olive oil, goose grease, goat butter and other lubricants have all been used at times; in parts of Africa a handful of oily dough is used to absorb dirt and toxins from the skin surface as the massage soothes the muscles.

Some oils are more pleasant and versatile than others, and have a beneficial effect on the skin in themselves. Probably the most useful oil, and the one most widely used in professional massage, is sweet almond oil. It is light, non-greasy and easily absorbed by the skin. Neutral and non-allergenic, it is even suitable for massaging babies. Grapeseed oil seems to suit oily skins quite well; it is reasonably priced and widely available. Rather thicker, but still a useful alternative, is soya oil.

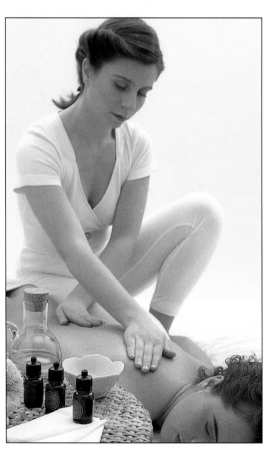

Sunflower oil may be used for massage if nothing else is available, though it may give a slight hint of salad dressing! Olive oil certainly does, although this was traditionally used in Mediterranean countries. Do not use mineral oils, such as baby oil: they sit on the surface of the skin and feel very greasy.

ENRICHING THE OIL BLEND

Other oils extracted from nuts or seeds all have their own particular qualities and, while they may be a little sticky and rich to use on their own for massage, they can be added to a lighter vegetable oil to create a mixture especially suitable for an individual skin type.

Walnut oil acts as a co-ordinator and balances the nervous system; like evening primrose oil, it can help to alleviate menstrual problems, including pre-menstrual tension. Sesame oil is ideal for stretch marks. Apricot kernel, peachnut and evening primrose oils are all good for cell regeneration and are particularly useful for face massage. Hazelnut oil is astringent and therefore good for oily skin, while jojoba benefits oily and sensitive skins and is valuable in the treatment of acne. For dry skins, a little wheat germ oil or avocado oil may be added.

These oils are all rich in nutrients, but when buying them, check that they have been naturally processed and not chemically treated. Cold-pressed oils are always the best.

Essential oils, blended into the base oil, will enhance the therapeutic effect of the whole massage experience with their own special properties and fragrance.

ESSENTIAL OILS

Essential oils may be added to the base oils, both for fragrance and for their therapeutic effects. By spreading evenly and easily over the skin, the massage oils encourage the quick absorption of the therapeutic oils into the skin.

Essential oils are highly concentrated and should be treated with respect: if in doubt, do not use them, and if any skin irritation occurs, wash the oil off immediately with warm water and a mild soap.

Always buy essential oils in dropper bottles, and dilute them safely for use on the skin. As a general rule, up to 5 drops of essential oil in 10 ml/2 tsp carrier oil is enough for a body massage. Never be tempted to use more essential oil than the amount recommended.

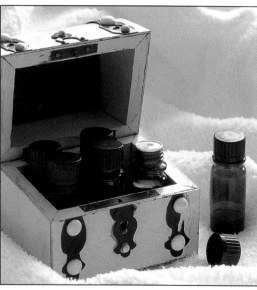

Store essential oils in their dropper bottles, in a cool, dry place and away from inquisitive children.

CAUTIONS: Essential oils are wonderful natural remedies for a variety of problems, and their aromatic effects can enhance mood, release tensions and reduce stress. But they are highly concentrated substances and must be used with caution. Follow the points listed below and, for the treatment of persistent problems, always ask the advice of a qualified aromatherapist. If in *any* doubt at all, seek a medical opinion before using essential oils.

• Never take essential oils internally, unless professionally prescribed.

• Do not use the same oils for more than one or two weeks at any one time in the treatment of specific ailments.

• When mixing your own blends, do not use more than three oils in any one treatment as the synergistic effects are less predictable.

• Do not use oils in pregnancy without first getting professional advice. The following oils are strongly contra-indicated at this time: bay, basil, cedarwood, clary sage, comfrey, fennel, hyssop, juniper, marjoram, melissa, myrrh, rosemary, sage and thyme.

• For anyone who has skin problems, test the diluted oil on a small area first. Dilute the oils even more than recommended, and if any skin irritation occurs, stop using the oils immediately. Do not use wheat germ oil on anyone who has an allergy to wheat. A few essential oils, such as bergamot, make the skin more sensitive to sunlight, and should be used with caution in hot, sunny weather.

• Be extra careful with anyone who has asthma or epilepsy. If they do experience a reaction, wash the oil off immediately.

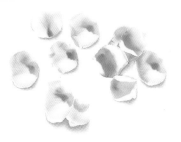

MIXING OILS FOR MASSAGE

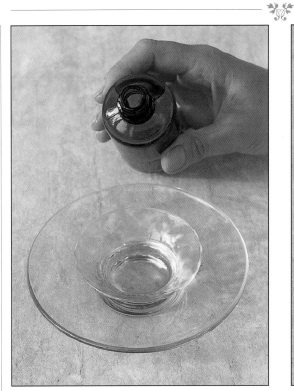

1 Assemble all the ingredients for your blend, but keep the essential oils covered until needed. Measure out your chosen base oil into a bowl.

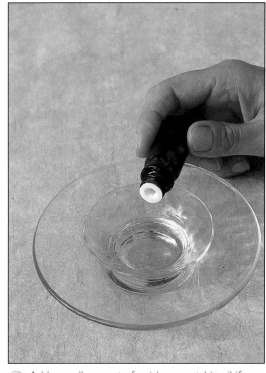

2 Add a small amount of a richer vegetable oil if you wish to make a blend to suit a particular skin type. Add the essential oil, one drop at a time, and mix gently to blend. Keep the oil covered during the massage to minimize evaporation of the essential oil.

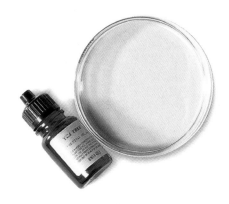

Adding an appropriate essential oil can heighten the effect of a massage considerably.

RECOMMENDED OIL BLENDS

For a generally relaxing massage blend, try essential oils of lavender and marjoram in equal amounts in a base vegetable oil. Both of these help to release tense, tired muscles and to induce a warm, relaxed glow. For a more invigorating, uplifting blend, add essential oils of bergamot and geranium to your massage oil. These have a refreshing effect on the whole system.

CHOOSING ESSENTIAL OILS

Essential oils may be extracted from exotic plants such as sandalwood or ylang ylang, or from more common plants like lavender and chamomile, but each one has its own characteristics and properties. The power of aromatics is quite subtle – as you get to know the different oils, you will come to understand their effects and learn which ones will blend well together. Never try to sniff a pure essential oil straight from the bottle, but place a single drop on the side of a glass.

Bergamot *(Citrus bergamia)*
This is the most effective antidepressant of all, best used at the start of the day. Do not use before going into bright sunlight, as it increases photosensitivity.

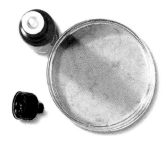

Bergamot

Black pepper *(Piper nigrum)*
The essential oil of black pepper is warming, comforting and sweet. It is very effective for poor circulation, aches and pains and stiffness.

Cedarwood *(Cedrus atlantica)*
The sweet, woody aroma of cedarwood oil has a calming effect. Use for skin complaints such as acne, alopecia, dandruff and eczema.

Chamomile *(Anthemis nobilis)*
Chamomile is relaxing and antispasmodic, helping to relieve tension headaches, nervous digestive problems and insomnia. It is also for useful and menstrual and menopausal problems.

Cypress *(Cupressus sempervirens)*
Astringent and antispasmodic, cypress can be used for circulatory problems, colds and coughs, menstrual problems and nervous tension. Do not use on anyone who suffers from high blood pressure.

Eucalyptus *(Eucalyptus globulus)*
One of the finest oils for respiratory complaints. Well diluted (never use more than 1 drop to 5 ml/ 1 tsp base oil), it can be applied to the forehead to relieve a hot, tense headache linked with tiredness. It has a cooling effect, reduces fever and is also a remedy for muscular or rheumatic aches and pains.

Geranium *(Pelargonium graveolens)*
The rose-scented geranium has useful properties, including its ability to bring a blend together for a more harmonious scent. Geranium has a refreshing, antidepressant quality, good for nervous tension, exhaustion, circulatory and skin problems.

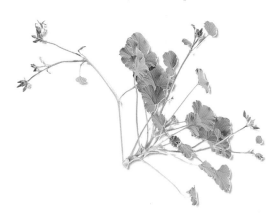

Geranium

Ginger *(Zingiber officinale)*
The essential oil of ginger is known for its balancing nature. It is helpful in cases of muscular aches and pains, poor circulation, coughs and colds, rheumatism, nausea and loss of appetite. The oil is comforting and grounding at the same time; it

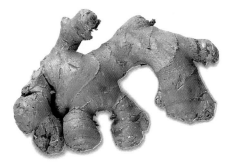

Ginger

can warm flat and cold emotions, and will sharpen the senses and memory. It blends well with citrus oils, neroli, rose and sandalwood, but should be used only in the lowest concentrations.

Jasmine *(Jasminum officinale)*
A favourite of the Arabs, Indians and Chinese, jasmine has a relaxing, euphoric effect. It can greatly lift the mood when there is debility, depression and listlessness. It will relieve menstrual cramps and is soothing to inflamed or irritated skin.

Juniper *(Juniperus communis)*
Juniper's most important use is as a detoxifier; it is effective for cellulite and in cases such as an absence of menstrual periods, cystitis, water retention and painful periods. Juniper should be avoided by people with kidney disease. It is uplifting and warming, and is known to be a helpful aid in coping with challenging situations.

Lavender *(Lavandula angustifolia/officinalis)*
One of the safest and most versatile of all essential oils, lavender has been used for centuries as a

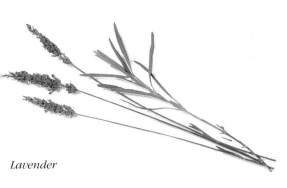

Lavender

refreshing fragrance and as a remedy for stress-related ailments. It is especially helpful for tension headaches or for nervous digestive upsets. Use in a blend for a deeply relaxing and calming experience.

Lemon (*Citrus limonum*)
Possibly the most cleansing and antiseptic of the citrus oils, lemon is useful for boosting the immune system and in skin care, when it is effective on oily skin. It can also refresh and clarify the thoughts. Like all citrus oils, it deteriorates quickly.

Marjoram (*Origanum majorana*)
Marjoram has a calming, warming effect, and is good for both cold, tight muscles and for tense people who suffer from anxiety headaches, migraines and insomnia. Use in massage blends for rubbing into tired and aching muscles, especially in the evening to encourage a good night's sleep. It blends well with bergamot, lavender and rosemary.

Neroli (*Citrus aurantium*)
Neroli is one of the finest of the floral essences. Its effect is uplifting and calming, bringing a feeling of

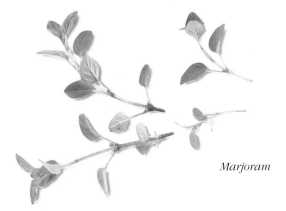

Marjoram

peace. It is useful during times of anxiety, panic, hysteria, shock and fear. It can help promote self-esteem and is particularly effective for nervous diarrhoea and other stress-related conditions.

Orange (*Citrus aurantium*)
Refreshing but sedative, orange is a tonic for anxiety and depression, having a similar effect to neroli, distilled from the blossom of the same plant. Orange also stimulates the digestive system and is effective for constipation. Because the oil oxidizes very quickly, it cannot be kept for very long.

Palmarosa (*Cymbopogon martini*)
Palmarosa was used to adulterate the highly prized rose oil known as attar of roses, gaining the name "Indian" or "Turkish" oil. This refreshing oil is gentle and comforting, and effective for skin inflammations, scars, weak digestion and headaches.

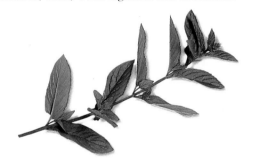

Peppermint

Peppermint (*Mentha piperita*)
Peppermint's analgesic and antispasmodic effects make it very useful for muscular aches and pains, sore feet, indigestion and flatulence, stomach cramps, nausea, colds and fevers. Diluted in a base oil, it can be rubbed on to the temples to ease tension headaches.

Rose (*Rosa* x *damascena trigintipetala*)
The scent evokes a general sense of pleasure and happiness. The actions of the oil are sedating, calming and anti-inflammatory. Not surprisingly, rose oil has a wide reputation as an aphrodisiac, and where anxiety is a factor it can be very beneficial. Add to a base massage oil to soothe muscular and nervous tension. It is particularly good for older, drier skins.

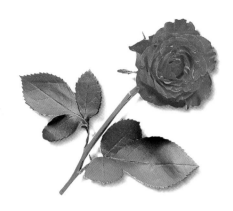

Rose

Rosemary (*Rosmarinus officinalis*)
With a very penetrating, stimulating aroma, rosemary has been used for centuries to help relieve nervous exhaustion, tension headaches and migraines. Rosemary stimulates the lymphatic system, improves circulation to the brain, and is an excellent oil for mental fatigue and debility. Avoid in cases of high blood pressure.

Sandalwood (*Santalum album*)
Probably the oldest perfume in history, sandalwood is known to have been used for over 4000 years. It has a relaxing, antidepressant effect on the nervous system, and where depression causes sexual problems, sandalwood can be a genuine aphrodisiac. Massage enhances its soothing effects.

Tea tree (*Melaleuca alternifolia*)
Tea tree oil is active against all types of infectious organisms; it is also a very powerful immune stimulant, increasing the body's ability to respond to these organisms. Its effect is cooling and refreshing, helping to clear the head. Vigorous and revitalizing, it is particularly useful after shock.

Ylang ylang (*Cananga odorata*)
This intensely sweet essential oil has a sedative yet antidepressant action. It is good for many symptoms of excessive tension, such as insomnia, panic attacks, anxiety and depression. It also has a good reputation as an aphrodisiac, through its ability to reduce stress levels. It blends well with bergamot, sandalwood and jasmine.

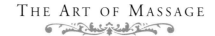

PREPARING FOR MASSAGE

Creating the right environment and space for treatment can contribute to making massage an even more relaxing and beneficial experience. Knowing that you are carefully prepared and in control will help your massage partner to relax completely. Your own state of mind is important, too, so take the time to compose yourself before you begin.

PREPARING THE ROOM

Before you start, make sure that the room is pleasantly warm and draught-free, and choose a quiet time when you will not be disturbed. If you are going to give the massage on the floor, pad the area with a thick layer of blankets or towels, or use a futon, so that your partner will be truly comfortable. It is not a good idea to massage on a bed, as the give of the mattress will counteract much of your effort.

Have plenty of freshly laundered towels ready to cover areas of the body that are not being worked on. If you are using oil, place it in a convenient spot where you can reach it easily without the risk of knocking it over.

PREPARING YOURSELF

Wear loose-fitting clothes for massage, ideally short-sleeved, with soft-soled, flat shoes, or work in bare feet. Take off your watch and any rings or bracelets, and make sure your nails are short. Take time to compose yourself so that your whole attention is focused on the massage. Try to do a few stretches and take some deep breaths to help you to feel calm; if you give a massage when you are tense yourself, this may be transmitted to your massage partner. This can work the other way round too, so feel prepared mentally to let go of any tensions that you feel coming from the other person's body and avoid absorbing these stresses yourself.

Give your partner privacy to undress, and clear directions on how to lie down on the mattress. Use the towels correctly to cover your partner's body. As well as keeping warm, a sense of modesty may be crucial to your partner's relaxation, and by following these suggestions, you will immediately make them feel safe and secure in your hands.

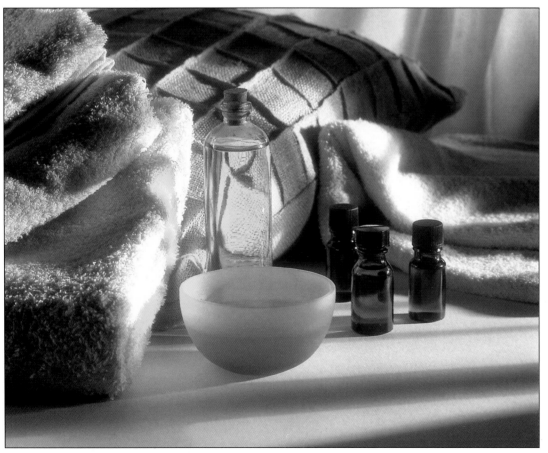

Freshly laundered towels, soft cushions and fragrant oils will all add to the comfort of your partner.

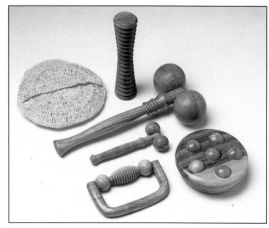

Instruments can play a useful role in self-massage.

MAKING CONTACT

Establish contact with your partner by placing your hands gently down on to the body, so that one hand rests on the top of the spine and the other at its base. Check that your own body is relaxed while giving your partner a few moments to settle into a comfortable position. When using oil, pour it on to your own hands first to warm it, never directly on to your partner's skin, as cold oil can cause an unpleasant shock – undoing the relaxing effect. Using smooth, flowing strokes, spread the oil slowly on to the skin, then begin the massage.

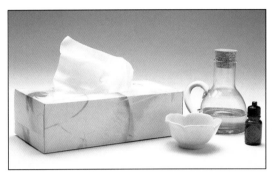

Make sure you have to hand everything you will need in the course of the massage, including a plentiful supply of tissues and the chosen oils.

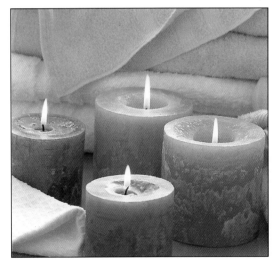

Candles and soft lighting will help create a mellow atmosphere and encourage relaxation.

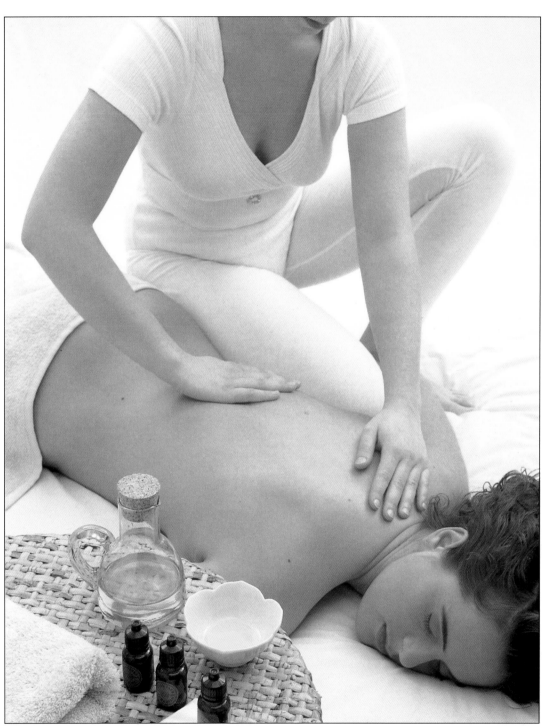

Making the initial contact is a key moment in the massage. The calm, unhurried way that you first touch your partner can lay the foundation for a soothing, unwinding experience.

BASIC STROKES

When many people think of massage they picture the vigorous pummelling and slapping often associated with puritanical health spas. In truth, firm massage can be highly beneficial without causing discomfort. Alternate firm and gentle flowing strokes to create a combination that will alleviate tension and muscular aches and pains while invigorating the body. There are four basic types of movement in Swedish massage: effleurage, petrissage, friction and tapotement.

EFFLEURAGE

Effleurage describes long, soothing, stroking movements, using the flat of the hand (or fingers if you are working on small areas). These strokes are often used to apply oil. You can use one hand on its own or with the other providing support on top of it, both hands at once or each hand alternately.

Effleurage is used to start off a massage, soothing the nerve endings and helping your partner to get used to your touch. It is used again at the end for a relaxing finish. In between, effleurage movements provide an important link between other, more stimulating strokes and are used to make first contact with a new area of the body. If you ever feel hesitant about what to do next, insert a few effleurage strokes to maintain continuity.

Repeat effleurage strokes several times. Each time, try to start the first complete stroke with light pressure, then apply slightly more pressure with the next complete stroke. Where there are large muscle areas, such as the thighs and back, you can apply the most pressure for a more stimulating effect.

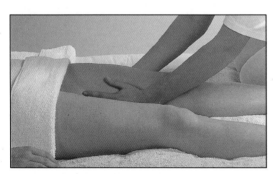

Relax the hands and mould them to the body. Use slow, continuous movements and keep your hands in contact with your partner between strokes.

CIRCLING

A movement allied to effleurage is circling, where the hands move large areas of muscle in a circular motion. Tension within muscles can produce knotted areas that may need working along or across the length of the fibres; this circular action starts to release the knots before deeper movements are used. It is essentially a slow, relaxing type of movement and should not be rushed.

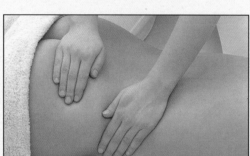

1 Lay both hands parallel to each other and flat on the area you intend to massage, keeping them about 10 cm/4 in apart. Circle both hands clockwise.

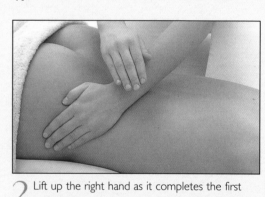

2 Lift up the right hand as it completes the first half-circle to allow the left hand to pass underneath it in an unbroken motion.

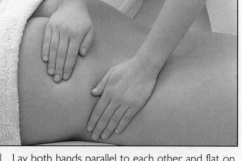

3 As the left hand continues to circle over the body, cross the right hand over it, dropping it lightly back on to the skin.

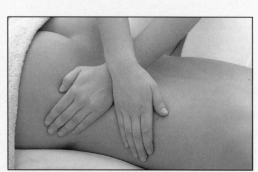

4 Let the right hand form another half-circle stroke before lifting off as the left hand completes its full circle. Repeat the sequence several times.

PETRISSAGE

A number of massage movements involve various ways of kneading, rolling and picking up the skin and muscles. These movements firm and strengthen the structures by stimulating the deep layers of tissue, increasing the supply of blood to the area and improving the flow of lymph. Generally, a single group of muscles, or an individual muscle, is worked on at one time. The basic kneading action is similar to kneading dough. With light kneading you are tackling the top muscle layers, while firmer kneading works further down, easing taut muscles and freeing congested tissues to eliminate waste products.

All muscular activity produces potentially toxic waste materials, notably lactic acid. If the person also gets tense and stiff, these wastes are trapped within the muscles, making them ache even more. Petrissage is a very effective way of encouraging the drainage of lactic acid and other waste matter, which in turn allows new blood to flow in, bringing oxygen and fresh nutrients to each cell.

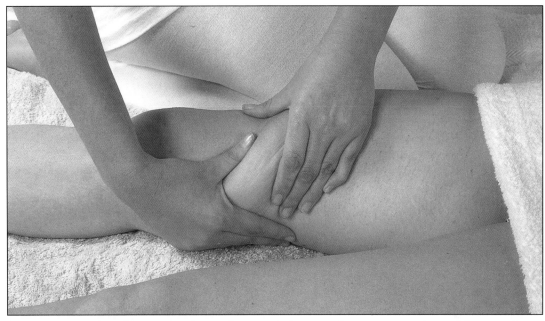

For petrissage, or kneading, start with your fingers pointing away from you, press down with your palm, grasp the flesh between fingers and thumb and push it towards the other hand. As you release the first hand your second hand grasps the flesh and pushes it back towards the first hand. It is a continuous action, alternating the hands to squeeze and release.

WRINGING

Another important petrissage-type movement is wringing, where the action of one hand against the other creates a powerful squeezing action in the muscles. When performed on the back, the person's own spine acts as a block against which the muscles are wrung. Make sure that your hands reach right round both sides of the body with each stroke, in order to get the most from the movement. Increase the speed of the stroke for an invigorating effect, then slow down towards the end for a soothing finish.

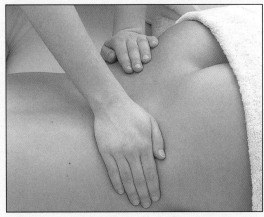

1 Place your right hand over the hip opposite to you and cup your left hand over the hip closest to you. Slide your hands towards each other with enough pressure to lift and roll the flesh on the sides of the body.

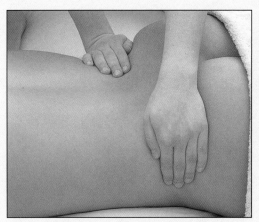

2 Decrease the pressure as you stroke across the back, hands passing each other to the opposite sides of the body. Without stopping, immediately begin to slide them back. Stroke your hands back and forth continuously while you wring up and down the lower back.

FRICTION

Friction, or "connective tissue massage", is a penetrating circular movement which applies direct pressure to a particular site of muscular tension, using the thumb, fingertips or knuckles. It is a valuable technique for concentrating on specific areas of tightness and muscle spasm in the back.

In general, pressure techniques are less painful when performed along the direction of the muscle fibres, rather than across them. Pressure is achieved by steadily leaning into the movement with the whole body, not by tensing your hands. The depth of the pressure applied should be adjusted for individual comfort; thinner people usually need lighter pressure and vice versa.

CAUTION: Do not attempt deep work if you are at all unsure of the effect, or if any pain occurs. Underdo rather than overdo the massage – effleurage and petrissage movements on their own can make a complete and thoroughly relaxing massage.

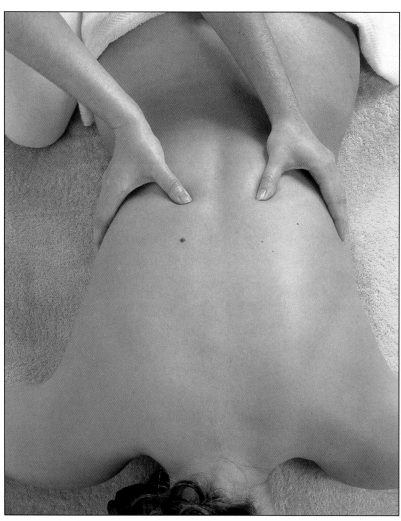

As you make the circular rotations you should actually feel the underlying tissues moving; you are not simply sliding over the surface of the skin.
A variation on circular friction is static pressure, where you lean gradually into the muscle, slowly deepening the pressure without the rotation action. Press for a few seconds, then gradually release.

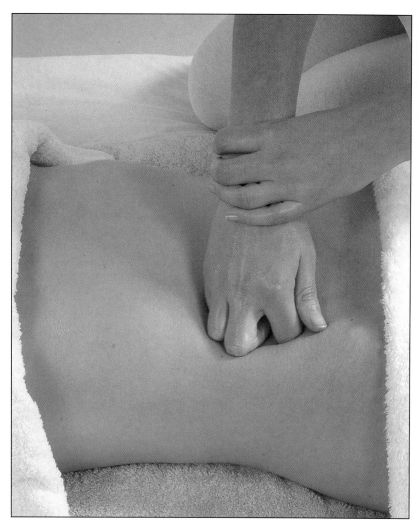

Another friction movement is knuckling: use the knuckles in a loosely clenched fist to produce rippling, circular motions. This movement is used to release tension up the sides of the spine and in other areas. Remember not to work directly over the spinal bone.

TAPOTEMENT

Tapotement, or percussion movements, are fast and stimulating. They include cupping, pummelling and hacking, which all sound like painful practices but which, when carried out properly, should certainly not cause bruising or pain. For all these movements, remember to keep your hands and wrists relaxed. All the percussion techniques are fast, precision actions, bringing one hand quickly after the other into contact with your partner. It is particularly important to ask your partner at the beginning whether you are applying the right degree of pressure.

These sequences stimulate the blood circulation, and also tone and help to strengthen sagging skin and muscles. In particular, they can tighten up areas of soft tissue, such as thighs and buttocks, which are prone to cellulite. Intersperse these brisk movements with gentler effleurage strokes.

CAUTION: Do not use percussion movements on particularly bony areas of the body as they will cause discomfort. As with all massage movements, never apply pressure on or below broken or varicose veins, only on the part of the leg which is higher than the vein (that is, closer to the heart).

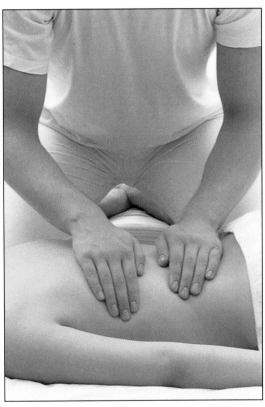

For cupping, gently curve the hands to make a loose cupped shape, bending at the knuckles while keeping the fingers firmly together. Do not bend the fingers too far over. Using the cupped palm, make a bouncy, brisk, cupping action against a fleshy area, alternating the hands quickly. The fast action creates a suction against the skin. Try this movement on the back, buttocks and thighs.

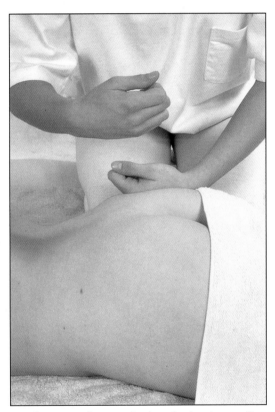

For the pummelling stroke, loosely clench your fists, but keep the wrists relaxed. You can make the strokes in two ways: either striking your partner with the outer edges of the loose fists, or with the front of the knuckles. Either way, the speed and rhythm of the movement is similar: brisk and firm, alternating the hands, without thumping your partner too enthusiastically. Once again, keep to the fleshier parts of the body, particularly cellulite zones such as hips, buttocks and thighs.

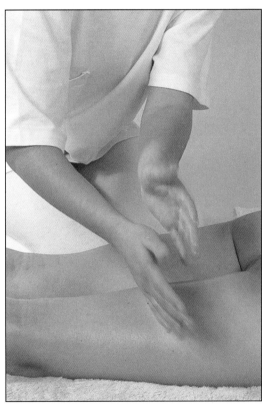

In hacking, the outer edge of the hand is used to stimulate the area by striking it quickly with alternate hands. You need to practise a brisk, bouncing movement, working rhythmically and rapidly over a fleshy area of the body. You need to have very relaxed wrists and fingers, and use the sides of the palm rather than the fingers. Used over the buttocks and thighs, hacking will help to tone up muscle and disperse excess fluid.

ELF-MASSAGE

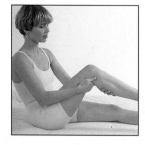

One of the nicest things about massage is that you do not need to invest in expensive equipment to perform the movements, and indeed several strokes can also be successfully used for self-massage. The advantage of working on your own muscles is that you will know exactly how deeply you can press, getting instant feedback from your body about the effects of the massage. Another benefit is that it helps you to practise the techniques and gain confidence before applying them to a partner. Obviously, it is not possible to do a complete massage on yourself, and therapeutically it cannot equal the experience of relaxing on a couch and surrendering yourself to an expert massage treatment. However, you will find that there are many times when you can help yourself if your body calls out for some physical work to relieve aching muscles.

Many activities inevitably lead to tensions in some part of the body, and regular quick massages can help both to ease these tensions and to prevent more chronic aches and pains. At any time of the day a short self-massage can help you to feel revitalized and reduce the impact of stress, both physical and mental. Follow these simple techniques whenever you are feeling stiff, aching or jaded, to de-stress your system and to help yourself look and feel better.

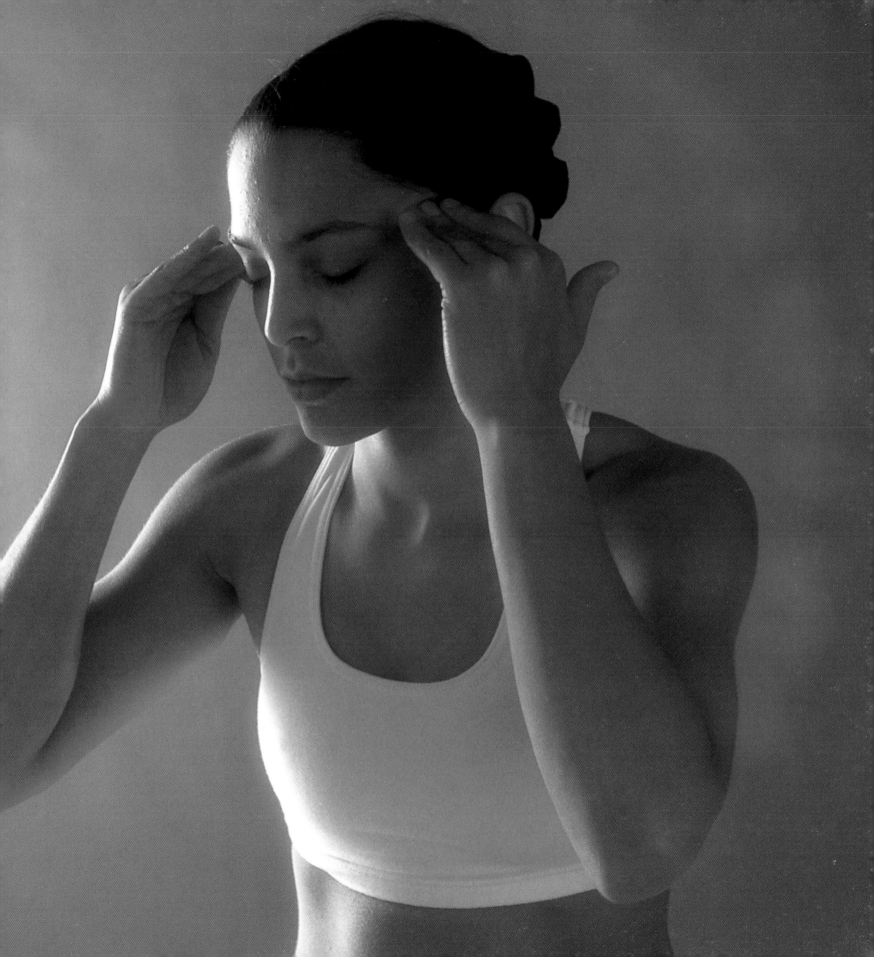

SHOULDERS

The build-up of tension and pain in the neck and shoulders are common symptoms of today's pressured and stressful work environments. Wherever you are, you can unknot tense muscles with these simple techniques.

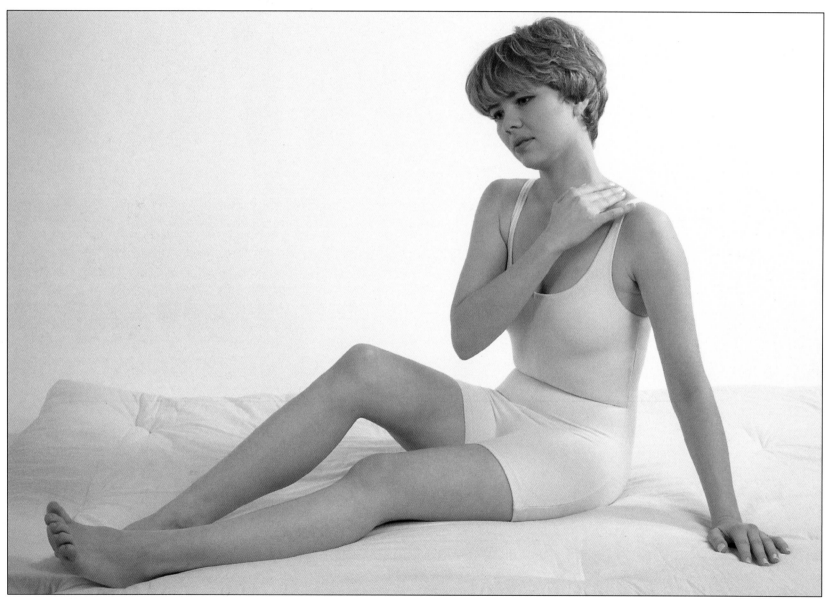

1 Sitting upright, start from the base of the neck and press down with your fingers along the top of the shoulders. As you reach the bony part of the shoulder, slide your hand back to the base of the neck, and repeat the pressing at least three times. Finish by stroking firmly from neck to shoulder and then repeat on the other side of the neck.

2 Use the fingertips of both hands to make small circular movements, working up the back of the neck. Gentle circular movements, where you can feel yourself easing muscular tightness, are better than direct, static pressures on this area. Continue up and round the base of the skull.

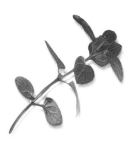

Peppermint essential oil works well for everyday aches and pains.

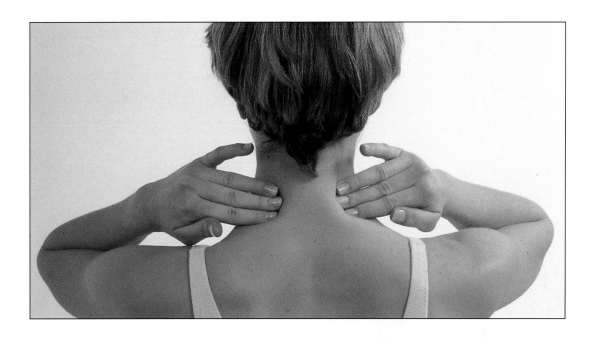

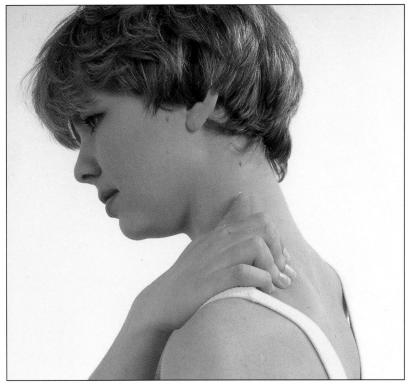

3 Knead each shoulder with a firm squeezing action, rolling the flesh between your fingers and the ball of your hand. Repeat several times on each side.

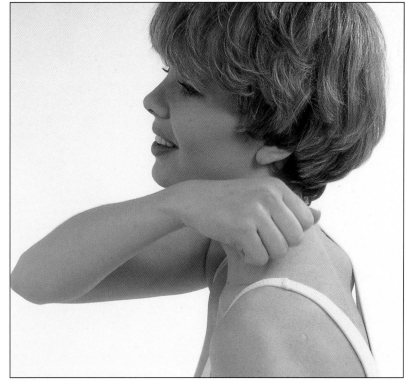

4 With your hand in a loose fist, pummel your shoulder lightly, keeping the wrist and elbow relaxed. Use light, springy movements to stimulate the area. Repeat on the other shoulder.

ARMS AND HANDS

Muscular tension forms in the arms and hands for a number of reasons. It may be a result of poor posture causing the shoulders to stiffen and leading to inflexibility in the arms, or may stem from repetitive movements at work which put strain on the muscles and tendons. Arm and hand massage is both relaxing and revitalizing.

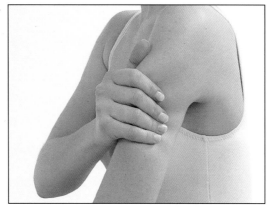

2 Pressing your fingers towards the palm of the hand, knead up the arm from the elbow to the shoulder. Cover the area thoroughly, working right around the arm.

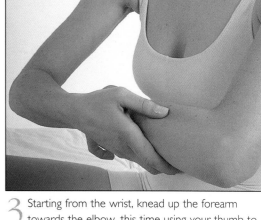

3 Starting from the wrist, knead up the forearm towards the elbow, this time using your thumb to make circular movements.

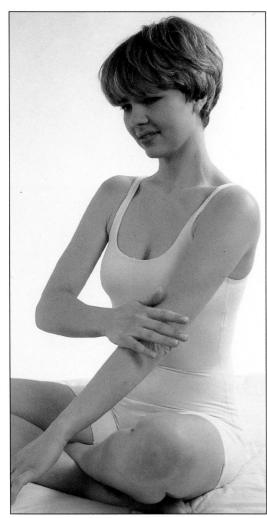

1 Stroke firmly up the arm from the wrist to the shoulder, returning with a lighter touch. Repeat the stroke several times on different parts of the arm.

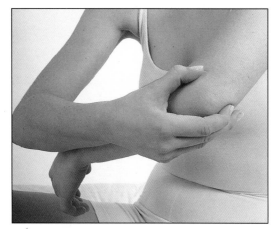

4 With thumb and fingers, make circular pressures around the elbow. First, work around the far side of the elbow with your working arm coming over the top of the arm you are massaging, then bend that arm up and work from the inside of your elbow. You may need to apply more oil for dry elbows.

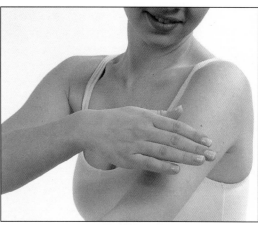

5 Gently but briskly pat your upper arm, or use some gentle cupping. Finish with some effleurage stroking up and down the whole arm again.

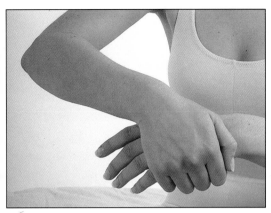

6 Squeeze the hand firmly, spreading the palm laterally. Cover the whole of the hand, fingers and wrist in this way.

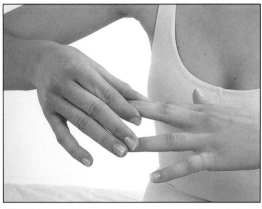

7 Using circular pressure, squeeze each finger joint between your finger and thumb. Then hold the base of each finger and pull the finger gently to stretch it, sliding your grip up to the top of the finger in one continuous movement.

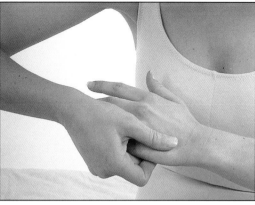

8 With circular thumb pressures, work up each of the furrows between the bones in the hand from the knuckle to the wrist. When you have covered each furrow, smooth the hand by stroking.

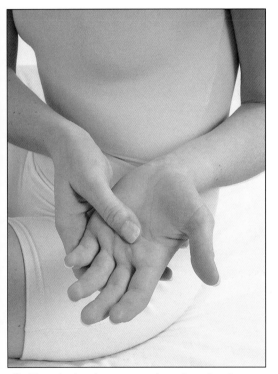

9 Turn the hand over to work on the palm. Cover the area with circular thumb pressures, paying particular attention to the heel of the hand and the wrist. Follow this with some deeper static pressures all over the palm.

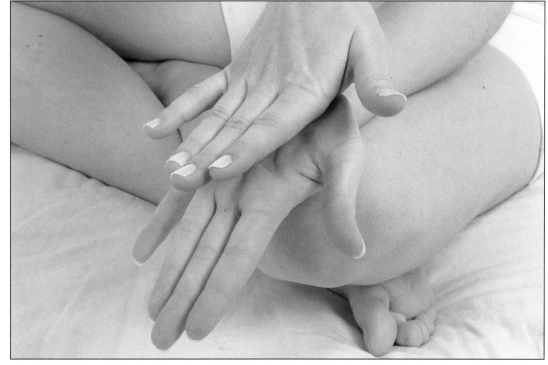

10 Finish by stroking the palm of one hand with the other. This can be quite a firm stroke, working from the tips of the fingers to the wrist, leading with the pressure from the heel of the hand. Stroke back to the fingers and repeat twice more, each time using slightly less pressure. Finally, stroke the inside of the wrist. Repeat the whole sequence on the other arm and hand.

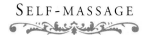

BACK AND ABDOMEN

Incorrect posture, long periods of standing or lifting heavy weights can all lead to pain in the lower back, while tension in the abdomen often reflects emotional unease and bottled-up feelings. A skilled, sensitive massage is the answer to both problems, but in the short term you may be able to relieve the discomfort a little with these techniques.

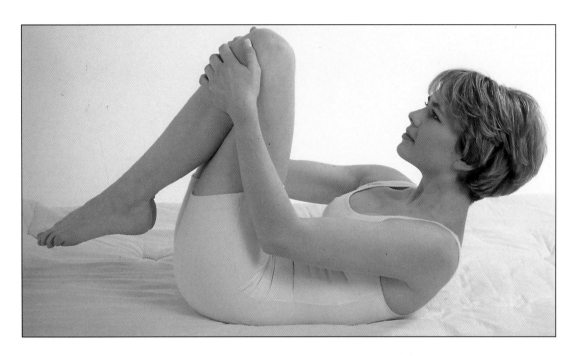

1 Lie on your back on the floor, clasp your knees and gently rock yourself backwards and forwards to massage the lower back, buttocks and hip joints, and gently stretch out the vertebrae.

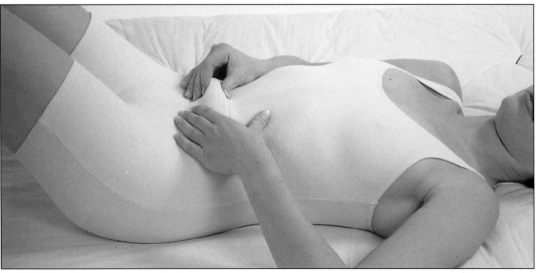

2 Bend your knees up and use some gentle petrissage to knead the whole of the abdominal area. When you have finished kneading, place both hands flat on the centre of the abdomen, fingers pointing slightly together, and pause for a few moments. Then smooth your hands outwards over the hips and thighs in one long, slow, moulding movement.

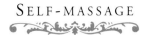

BUTTOCKS, HIPS AND THIGHS

If you have an accumulation of cellulite in these areas, a quick daily massage using percussion and kneading movements will help to shift fatty deposits under the skin.

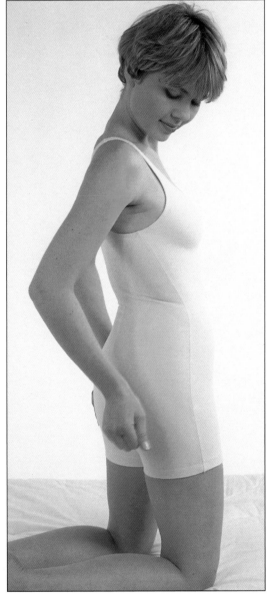

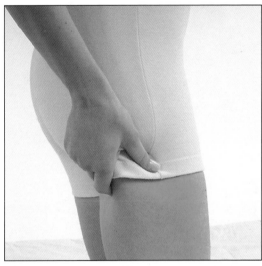

2 With the thumb and fingers, squeeze and release the muscles firmly and slowly, working from the top of the thigh over the buttock. Repeat the same movements on the other side.

3 Use both hands to squeeze and release the muscles on the front and side of the thigh, kneading the entire upper leg. Repeat on the other side.

4 Starting at the knee, stroke up the thigh with both hands to soothe the leg.

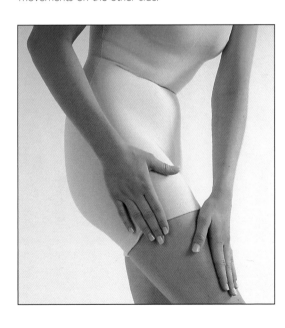

1 Kneel up and pummel your hips and buttocks, using a clenched fist. Keep your wrists flexible.

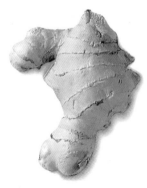

The essential oil of ginger will boost a sluggish circulation and help in the fight against cellulite.

LEGS AND FEET

Stroking and kneading movements will warm and stretch the large muscles of the legs, easing away tension, improving the circulation of blood and lymph and freeing contracted joints. Work through the whole sequence on one leg and foot before repeating it on the other side.

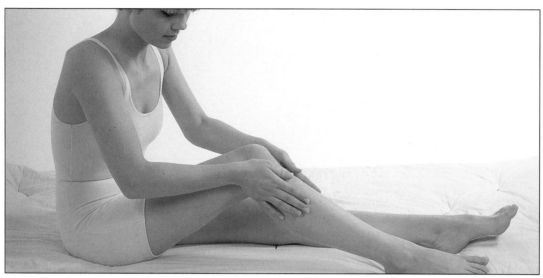

1 Sitting down on the floor, with one knee bent slightly, stroke the leg with both hands from ankle to thigh in one long continuous movement. Begin the stroke as close to the ankle as you can reach. Repeat several times, moving around the leg slightly each time to stroke a different part. Try to establish a rhythm for the strokes which you can maintain throughout the whole sequence.

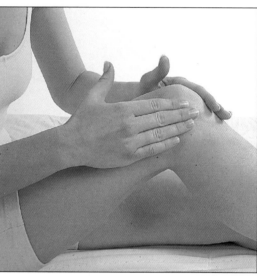

2 Massage the knee, stroking around the outside of the kneecap to begin with, then using circular pressure with the fingertips to work around the kneecap more firmly.

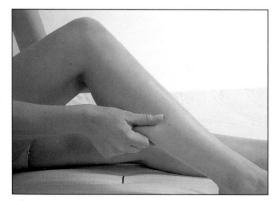

3 Knead the calf muscle with both hands, using a firm petrissage movement to loosen and release any tension in the muscle.

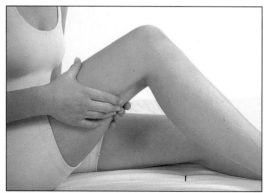

4 Continue kneading on the thigh, working over the top and outside areas with alternate hands. While the leg is still raised, do some soothing effleurage strokes up the back of the leg from ankle to hip.

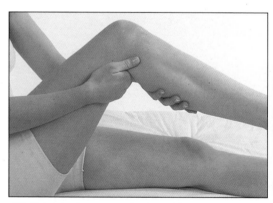

5 Raise the leg, supporting its weight with your hands under the knee. Rotate the ankle five times in each direction.

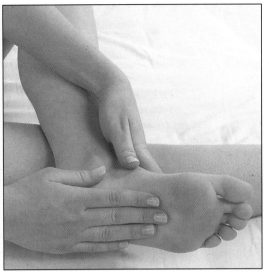

6 Gently bring your foot over the other leg. With one hand on top of the foot and one underneath, stroke up the foot from toes to ankle. Repeat the action three times.

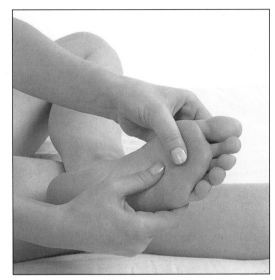

7 With the thumbs, apply circular pressure over the ball of the foot. Work in lines from the inside of the foot to the outer edge. Repeat three times.

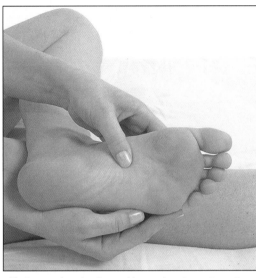

8 Supporting the foot with one hand, continue the circular pressures over the raised instep, working from the inner to the outer edge. Repeat three times.

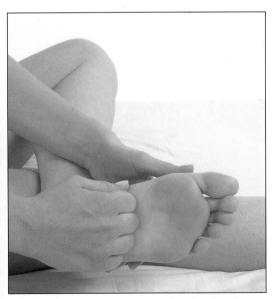

9 Still holding the foot with one hand, make a loose fist with the other and firmly rotate your fist over the instep. Work thoroughly into the arch.

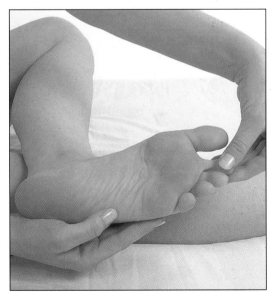

10 Massage each toe individually. Slowly stretch the toe between the thumb and finger: pull gently, moving your fingers up the toe each time, until you reach the tip.

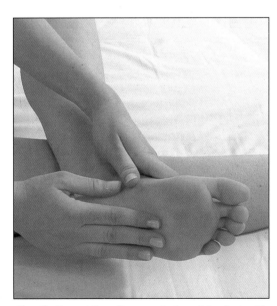

11 Repeat the effleurage strokes of the foot, with one hand over and one under the foot, working from toes to ankle several times.

Massage with a Partner

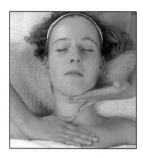 Probably the best way to improve and deepen a relationship is to increase caring physical contact, and massage is an ideal approach. The ability to ease tensions and deeply relax your partner is a very satisfying form of giving. Helping someone to release tension and feel better does not have to be limited to your life partner of course; there are other members of the family, friends or colleagues who can all be helped in this way, and a better rapport will be developed with them, too.

Being massaged by someone else means that you can let go of your muscles completely. It does require trust to do so, and if you are massaging a person you do not know too well, be sensitive to this. Massage practitioners are well aware that they are being given permission to make a deep contact with their clients, and that this is a privilege that must not be taken for granted.

Make sure that you have created the right environment for a truly relaxing massage. Check that your partner is warm and comfortable and take a few moments to make contact and accustom them to your touch before you begin. Do not press harder than is comfortable for your partner and, of course, take great care never to inflict pain while you are massaging, at any time.

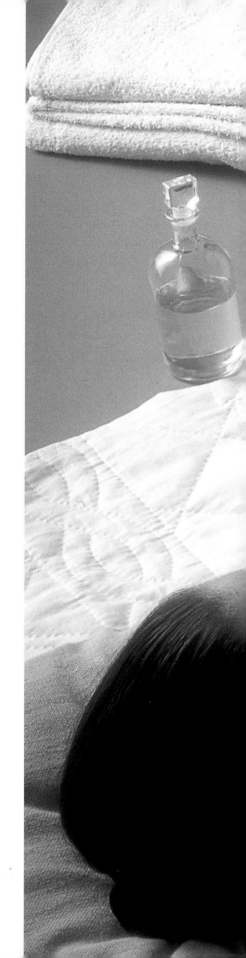

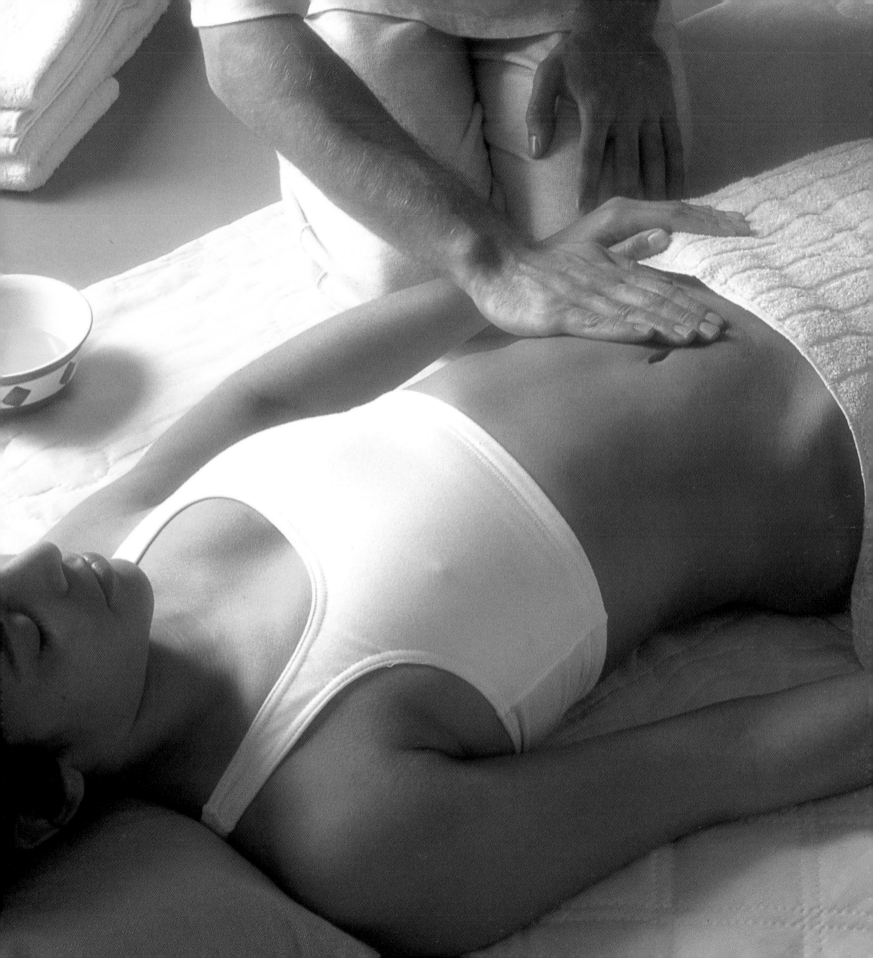

WHOLE BODY MASSAGE

A successful massage benefits and relaxes both body and mind, and careful preparation helps you to achieve this aim. Creating a nurturing ambience, preparing all your equipment and oils, and approaching the session in a calm and relaxed manner will give you confidence in your abilities and inspire trust in your partner.

The sequence shown on the following pages is a comprehensive, top-to-toe massage based on Swedish techniques and adapted for home practice. As a beginner you may find the full sequence too tiring at first. Until your hands and wrists build up their strength and you get used to positioning your own body comfortably to perform the massage, it is best to work on just a few parts of the body, such as the back of the legs, back and shoulders, or to perform fewer movements on each part of the body.

Your partner will find it more relaxing if you perform one or two types of movement thoroughly, rather than changing the strokes after a few seconds to cover all the steps. Always include effleurage strokes to begin and end a sequence, and never leave the body unbalanced – if you work on one leg or arm, you should repeat the same movements on the other side of the body.

Exchanging a regular basic massage is a luxury for both giver and receiver. However, you should not attempt to remedy specific problems: if in any doubt at all, seek the advice of a doctor or trained practitioner before you begin.

Pour a little oil into your palms at the beginning of the massage and oil your hands lightly again as you begin each new sequence of movements. You may need to replenish the oil more frequently if you are working on areas of very dry or hairy skin.

Establish contact with your partner by placing your hands on their body, and begin the massage with some smooth and flowing effleurage strokes.

> ### THE FULL MASSAGE SEQUENCE
> ❧
>
> **The front of the body**
> 1 Legs
> 2 Feet and ankles
> 3 Arms and hands
> 4 Chest, shoulders and neck
> 5 Face
> 6 Abdomen and waist
> **The back of the body**
> 7 Legs and buttocks
> 8 Back and shoulders

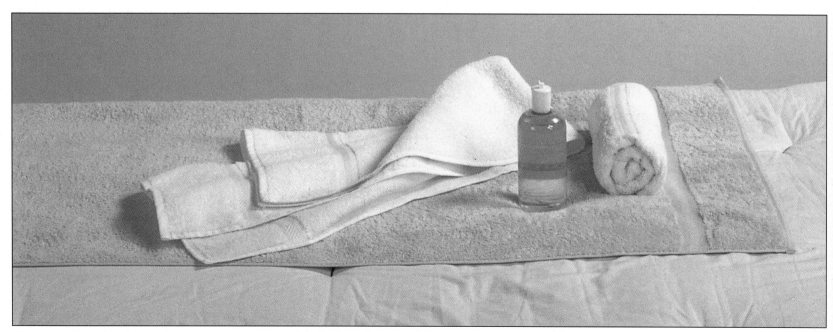

Have several towels ready, so that you can cover areas of the body not being worked on. A rolled towel behind your partner's neck or knees is often helpful.

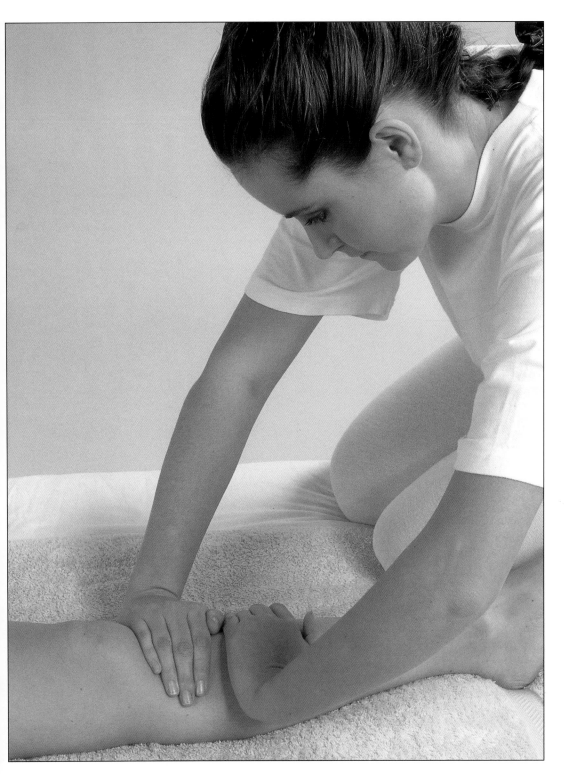

YOUR POSTURE AND BREATHING

A good posture will help you to perform fluid strokes and remain relaxed throughout the session, without straining your own body. Maintain a good, firm balance whether you are kneeling or standing, using your leg muscles to ease your body back and forth with your strokes. Keep your knees relaxed and your spine straight. Remind yourself to relax your shoulders and let your arms hang loosely so that your shoulders, elbows and wrists are flexible at all times. Keep a space between your arms and your body to avoid hunching your shoulders.

Deep and easy breathing will replenish your energy, allow tense muscles to open and relax, and bring vitality to your strokes. Synchronize your breath with your strokes to deepen the effects of your massage.

CAUTIONS: Never massage directly on top of the spine, though working down each side of the bony spinal column is fine, and produces many benefits.

There are occasions when giving a massage is not appropriate. Avoid massaging anyone suffering from any of the following conditions:
- heart condition
- high blood pressure
- bacterial or viral infection
- nausea or abdominal pain
- severe back pain which may originate in the spine, especially if there are shooting pains in any of the limbs
- temperature or fever
- open wound or skin infection
- cancer
- post-operative recovery

If you are in any doubt at all, it is always best to check with a doctor.

Pay attention to your posture as you perform the massage. By maintaining a balanced and relaxed position, you will avoid straining your own body.

THE FRONT OF THE BODY

The full massage begins with the front of the body, so your partner should lie face up with cushions or rolled towels behind the head and neck, and wherever they are needed for support.

THE LEGS

Since legs carry the full body weight, the bones and muscles in the legs are the largest and strongest we have. A good leg massage not only helps to relieve strain and tension in the legs themselves, but can benefit the well-being of the whole body. It's not unknown for backache to be traced to problems in the legs, and for a good leg massage to help alleviate the pain.

Leg massage stimulates the circulation of blood and lymph, and done regularly it helps to prevent varicose veins. Any congestion in the lower legs will be lessened with effleurage movements taken up toward the lymph nodes at the back of the knee and in the groin. If legs feel puffy or swollen to the touch, use only the gentlest of pressure.

Complete the whole sequence of movements on one leg and foot before moving around your partner to work on the other side.

CAUTION: You will need to take certain precautions if your partner has varicose veins. Never knead or put any pressure on varicose veins, and only massage the part of the leg higher than the area with the vein (that is, closer to the heart); never massage on or below the vein.

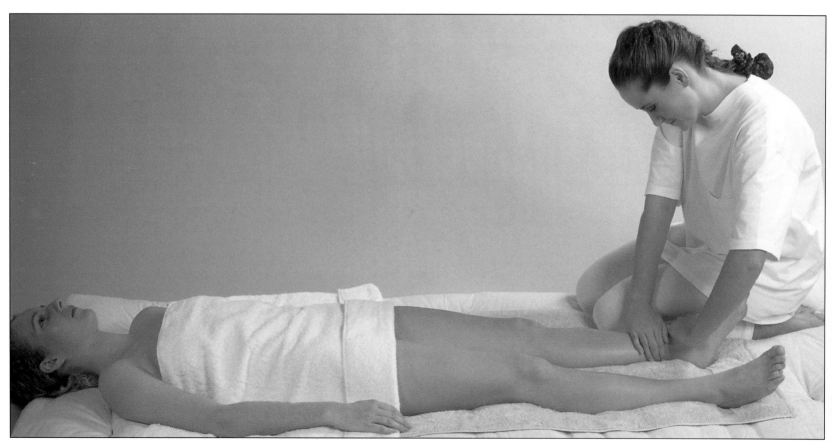

1 Kneel beside your partner's left ankle. Start with your hands crossed over the ankle, in readiness to begin several long effleurage strokes. You will need more oil if the legs are particularly hairy or dry, but don't add too much in the first instance.

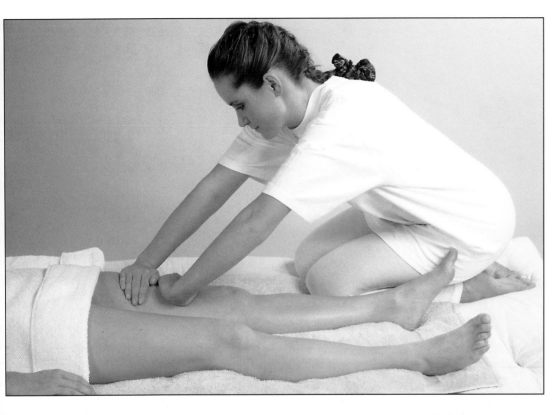

2 Keeping your hands crossed over the leg, slide the palms up the front of the leg, over the knee and up to the thigh, in one long, continuous, sweeping movement to oil the front of the leg evenly.

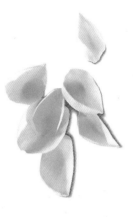

Rose oil is one of the most effective for promoting an overall feeling of well-being.

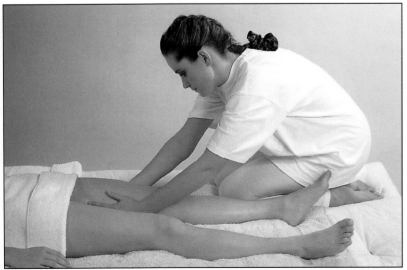

3 Turn the hands outwards around the hip, separate them and bring them back down each side of the thigh.

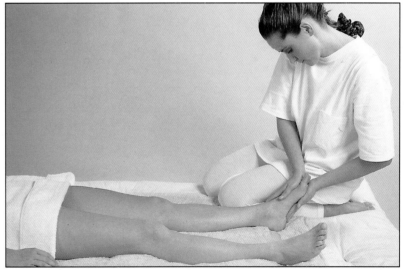

4 Continue to sweep the hands back to the ankle, and then over the foot to the toes. Then place your hands crossed over the ankle again, ready to repeat the entire movement. Use some more oil if necessary, and this time use slightly firmer pressure on the upward stroke, then lighter again for the return. The stroke is smooth and continuous throughout. Repeat the sequence over the whole leg once again.

THE THIGHS

Firm massage on the larger muscles around the thighs can dispel tiredness and stimulate a sluggish lymphatic system, which brings many health and vitality benefits.

THE KNEES

Move smoothly down the thigh to the knee, where you need to work very gently over the bony area.

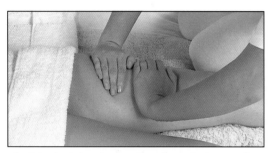

1 Bring both hands up to just above the knee and move them up together, pressing the muscles firmly towards the upper thigh. You should be applying enough pressure to see movement in the muscles.

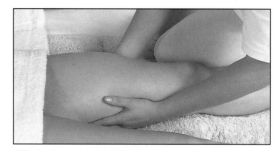

2 At the top of the thigh, separate the hands and, using lighter pressure, come down either side of the leg to the knee.

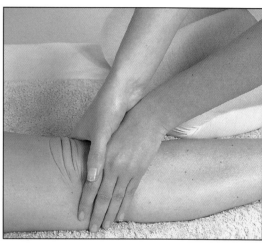

1 Place both hands just below the knee. Lightly massage around the kneecap, using your fingertips to work gently into the muscles around the bone. Maintain the massage for about 2 minutes.

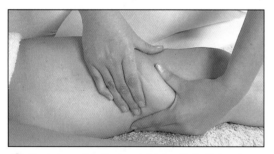

3 Begin kneading the inner thigh with both hands. Squeeze, then release the muscles, picking up and rolling them as you do so. Continue the kneading action over the top and outer thigh.

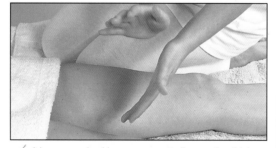

4 Now use a hacking movement all over the thigh area. Briskly strike the area with the outside edge of your hands, one hand after the other, using short, sharp, quick movements.

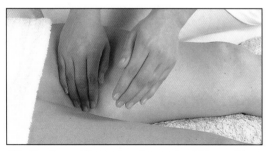

5 Continue with cupping all over the thigh, working quickly. Expect quite a loud cupping sound, but remember to check with your partner that the strokes are not too powerful.

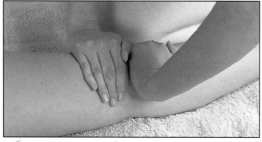

6 Beginning at the knee, do some effleurage strokes up to the top of the thigh, sweeping the hands outwards and back down to the knee, to soothe the area after the series of stimulating movements.

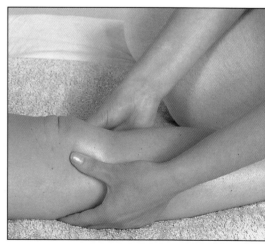

3 Support the back of the knee with your hands and use your thumbs to circle gently around the kneecap, working downwards. Return to the top of the knee and repeat three times.

THE CALVES

When you have finished working on the knee, do some more effleurage strokes, sweeping them up from the ankle to just below the kneecap and back down to the ankle, and repeating them several times.

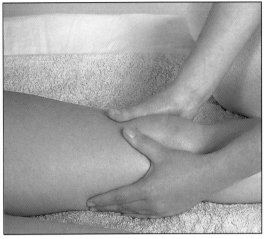

2 Starting with your thumbs above the kneecap, and with your hands under the knee for support, slowly draw them around the outside of the kneecap and release. Repeat this movement three times.

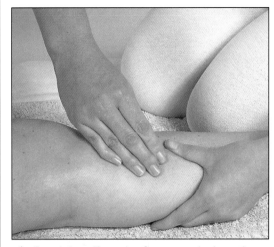

1 Knead the calf muscles. Squeeze and release them, working from the ankle up to the knee.

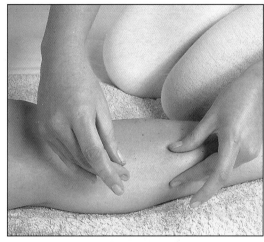

2 Lightly and quickly pinch the fleshy part of the calf with the fingers and thumbs, one hand after the other. Check with your partner that you are not pinching too hard; although it does need to be felt to be effective, this should not actually be painful.

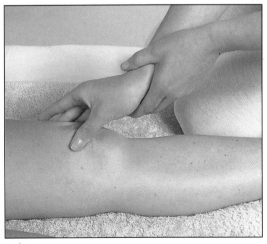

4 Raise the height of your hands above the knee. Work around the kneecap with one hand, loosening the muscles with your thumb and fingers. Use gentle circular rotations to cover the area thoroughly. You may find it easier to support your wrist with the other hand, to prevent your wrist from becoming tired.

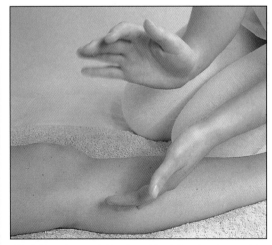

3 Using the outside edge of both hands, alternately and rhythmically strike the calf muscles, working up and down the entire length of the lower leg, but keeping away from the back of the knee and the bony shin area. Keep the hacking action short and brisk.

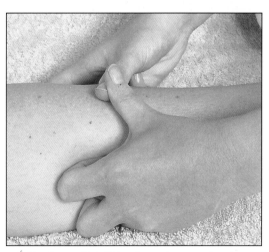

4 Starting at the ankle and crossing your thumbs on top of the shin for support, make semicircular kneading movements with loose knuckles, working up and down the calf. Finish with some relaxing effleurage movements from ankle to thigh.

THE FEET AND ANKLES

A foot massage is particularly relaxing after the legs have been worked on. It can alleviate anxiety and stress, stimulate the circulation and nervous system, promote sleep and energize anyone feeling tired and lethargic. There are thousands of nerve endings in the foot, especially on the sole. Try to include the ankles too, to improve their flexibility.

Change the pressure of the strokes to suit your partner, remembering that deeper pressure tends to revitalize, whereas gentle strokes increase relaxation. When working on the feet it is best to use only a very little oil, otherwise your hands will slide around and tickle. If your partner's feet are hot and sticky, use a little talcum powder instead.

Before starting, you may wish to raise the knee slightly with a rolled towel, to relax the muscles around the knee and in the lower back.

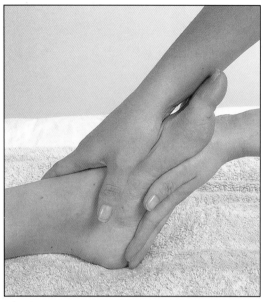

1 Kneel at your partner's feet. Starting with your hands at the ankle, gently slide them towards the tips of the toes and then release them. Repeat several times. If you are using oil, apply it with this stroke.

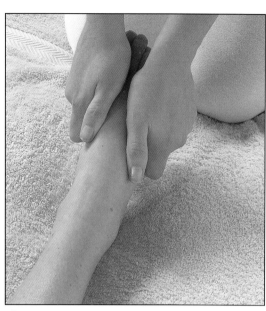

2 With the heels of your hands, give a good stretch to the top of the foot. Draw the hands towards the sides of the foot to give the stretch. Repeat a few times, working slightly further down the foot.

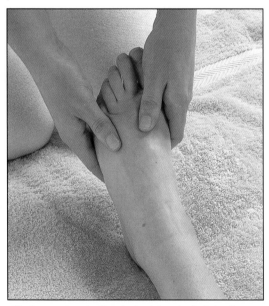

3 Supporting the foot in both hands, find the furrow between each tendon and, using small circular movements, work both thumbs up the tendons towards the ankle. Repeat three times on each tendon.

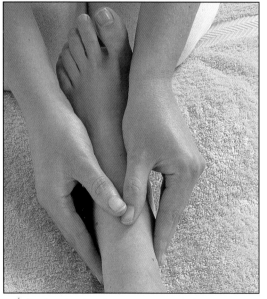

4 Resting the thumbs across the top of the ankle, work the fingers right around the ankle bone, using light, circular movements.

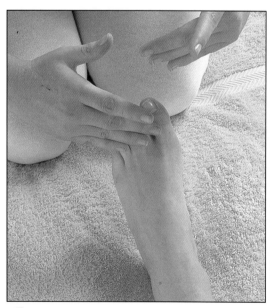

5 Lightly tap the toes with your fingers to build up some gentle friction.

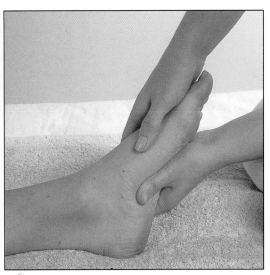

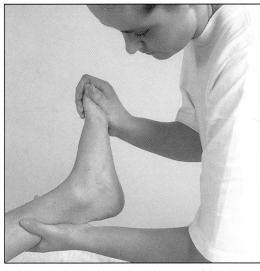

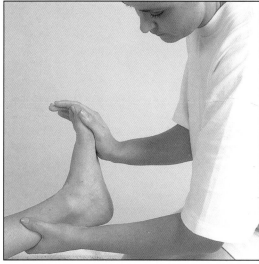

6 Knead the foot firmly, working particularly well into the arch. You will need to use different parts of the hand, such as the heel, knuckle and thumbs.

7 Supporting the lower leg with your left hand, gently rotate the ankle three times in each direction, without forcing it.

8 Give the foot a gentle stretch backwards and forwards, to relax and flex the tendons. Supporting the back of the lower leg, use your other hand at the toes to push the foot gently away from you. To reverse the stretch, take the hand over the top of the foot and press the foot down, still supporting the lower leg with the other hand.

9 Finish the foot and ankle sequence with some long sweeping effleurage strokes from the top of the foot up the lower leg and back down to the foot, to help reintegrate the foot and the leg. Repeat several times, varying the pressure.

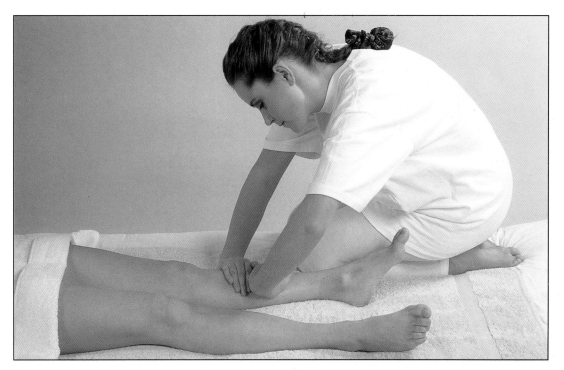

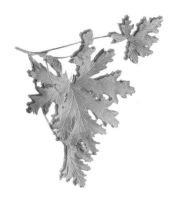

The oil extracted from the geranium plant has stimulating and uplifting properties.

THE ARMS

Arms and hands can hide the most powerful emotions. Tight, clenched arms and hands often reflect insecurity, self-protection and unresolved anger. Whether the posture is intentional or subconscious, tension in the arms can cause headaches, neck pain and aching shoulders. Don't be put off if your partner's arms are slim and bony; there are still important muscle areas there.

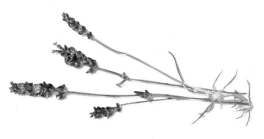

Mellow and peaceful lavender oil has been valued for centuries for its calming qualities.

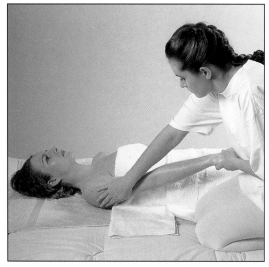

1 Kneel halfway along your partner's right side. Holding the wrist with your left hand, lightly oil the arm using effleurage strokes, starting from the wrist and sweeping your hand up around the shoulder and down again. Repeat three times.

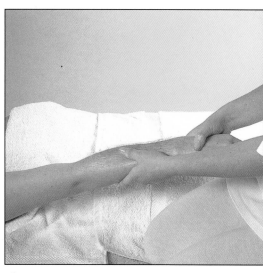

2 Changing hands, so that your partner's wrist is supported in your right hand, use the left hand to stroke gently from the wrist to the shoulder, and back down again. Repeat several times.

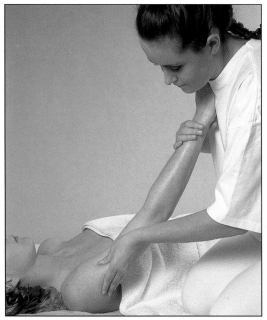

3 Lift the arm and rest the hand on your right shoulder ready to start kneading. Support your partner's wrist with your right hand and use your left hand to knead the muscles of the upper arm lightly.

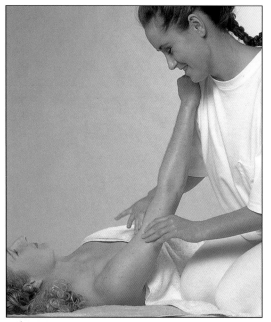

4 Keeping your partner's hand supported by your shoulder, use the fingers of both hands to continue the kneading.

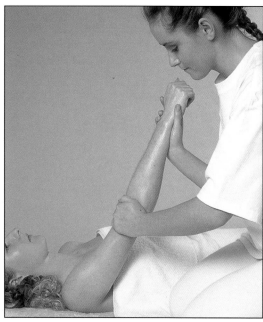

5 Still holding the arm across the front of your chest with your right hand, do some effleurage strokes from the elbow up to the shoulder and back down again. Repeat three times.

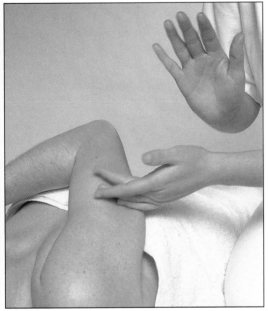

6 Bend your partner's arm and rest the right hand on the left shoulder. Using the outside edges of your hands, do some short, brisk hacking on the outer and under sides of the arm.

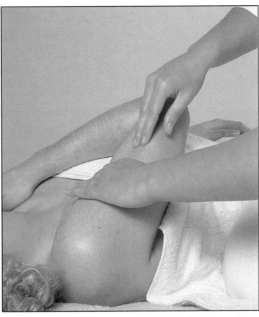

7 With your partner's arm still bent, firmly knead the muscles of the upper arm with your right hand, using the left hand to keep your partner's arm stable.

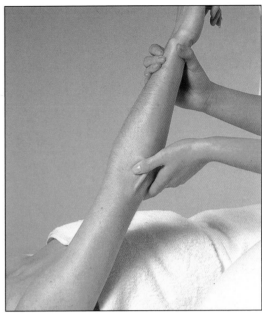

8 Holding the wrist for support with your right hand, work around the outside of the elbow with your fingers and thumb, using smooth circular movements and covering the area thoroughly. As the elbows can get very dry, you may need some more oil.

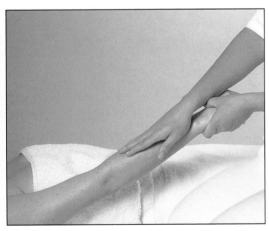

9 To encourage further relaxation, hold the wrist with your left hand and do some effleurage strokes up and down the top of the forearm. Keep the pressure fairly firm.

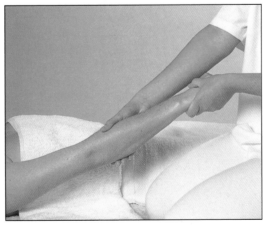

10 Repeat these effleurage strokes on the inside of the forearm.

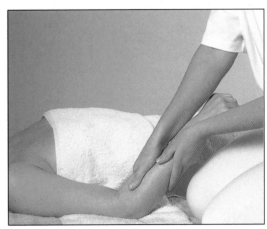

11 Rest your partner's elbow back on the towel. Supporting the weight of the lower arm in your left hand, use your right hand to knead the inside of the forearm, starting from the wrist. When you reach the elbow, glide gently back to the wrist to begin again. Repeat three times. Finish the arm with a few effleurage strokes.

THE HANDS AND WRISTS

A hand massage is surprisingly effective, and is almost on a par with having the feet massaged. Our hands are in almost constant use throughout the day, at work, for household chores or in leisure activities, acting simultaneously as multi-purpose tools and shock barriers. Not surprisingly then, a lot of tension creeps into the hands, and a massage is a reminder of how good it feels to relax them completely. Massaging the arms and hands increases suppleness and dexterity, and can liberate and relax not only the muscles but also the pent-up emotions, as your partner starts to feel the wonderful sensation of letting go.

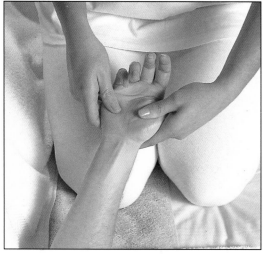

1 Support your partner's hand in both hands and gently use the thumbs to knead the palm. This should be a continuous, circular action, with the thumbs alternately applying the pressure.

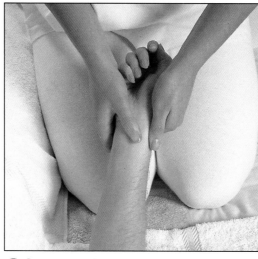

2 Rest your hands under your partner's wrist and use the thumbs to stroke outwards around the wrist. Then work with the thumbs up the inner forearm toward the elbow, using circular movements.

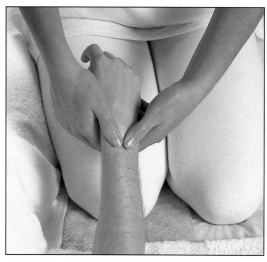

3 Turn your partner's hand over, supporting the wrist with one hand. Massage over the back of the wrist with your thumbs, taking care to keep the movements light as you work over the bone.

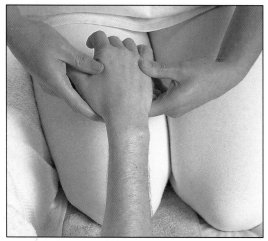

4 Stroke up in between the tendons on the back of the hand with your thumbs, from knuckles to wrist, using light, small circles. Repeat twice between each tendon.

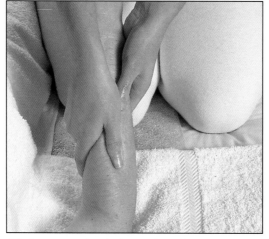

5 Sweep your hands alternately up from the wrist towards the elbow, applying a fairly firm pressure with the inside edge of the hands. Repeat several times.

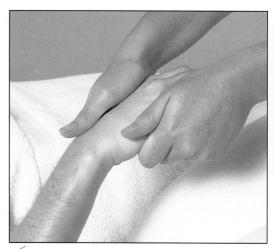

6 Come back down to the hand and gently stretch the back of the hand, drawing your own hands out towards the sides.

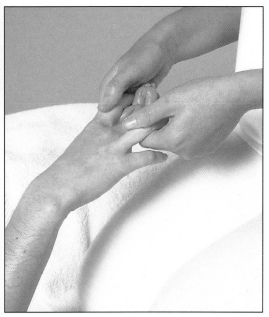

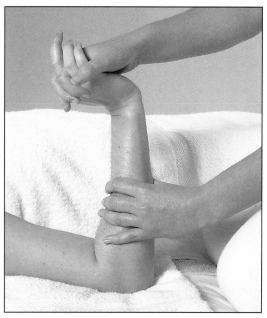

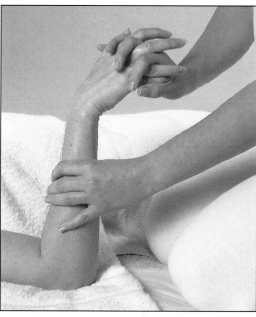

7 With one hand, make circular pressure movements around the finger joints, starting at the tip. When you have worked around all joints, rotate each finger twice. Stretch each finger to release the joints.

8 Raising your partner's lower arm and supporting it with your left hand, clasp your partner's hand with your right hand and gently rotate it in a half-circle, three times in each direction.

9 Still supporting the lower arm, thread your fingers between your partner's and gently bend the wrist backwards and forwards three times, making sure that the wrist joint is not forced.

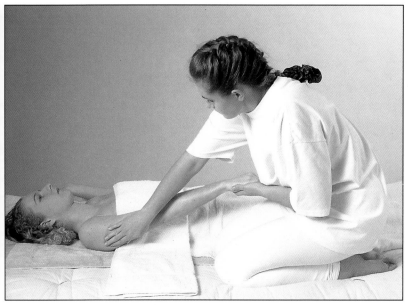

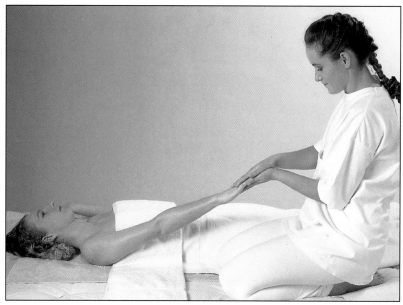

10 Finish the arm and hand sequence by stroking the entire length of the arm and hand with some soothing effleurage from palm to shoulder.

11 Hold your partner's hand between both of your palms for several seconds, then release, lowering the arm gently. Move around to kneel on the other side and repeat the arm and hand massage on the left.

THE CHEST

It's not only the hours spent sitting hunched over a desk that tighten and contract the chest muscles – emotional tension is often stored in the chest area, and clutching a car steering wheel, carrying heavy shopping and poor posture all have a cumulative effect.

Before you begin, check whether your partner's neck would be more comfortable with a small cushion or folded towel under the head. Kneel behind your partner's head to start the sequence.

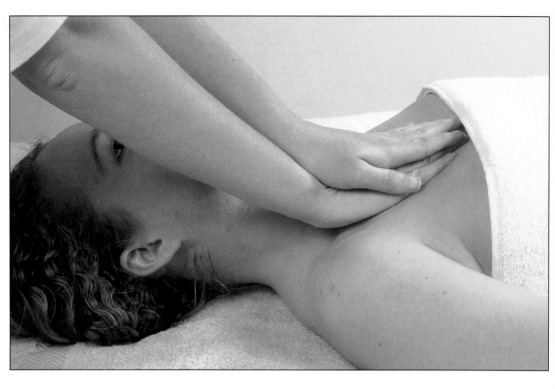

1 With the flat of the hands placed on the chest, fingers pointing away from you, place your left hand on top of the right. You will be doing reinforced effleurage on the right side of the chest first.

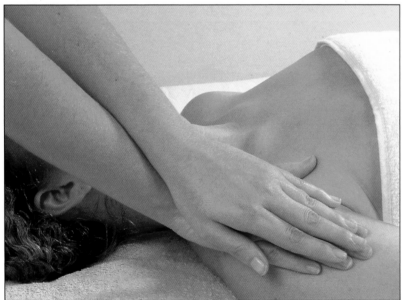

2 Sweep your hands over the chest, towards and around the right shoulder, keeping the left hand over the right, in a continuous effleurage stroke. You should apply enough pressure to press the chest and shoulder towards the floor, so that they release as you end the stroke. Repeat three times.

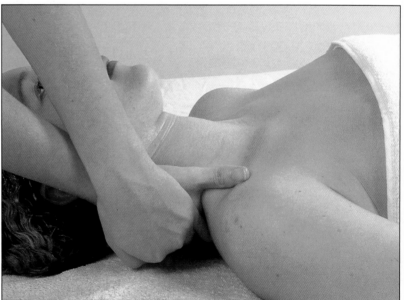

3 Continue the effleurage stroke, sweeping both hands around and up the right side of the neck. Repeat the sequence twice more, starting from the centre of the chest each time, as in step 1.

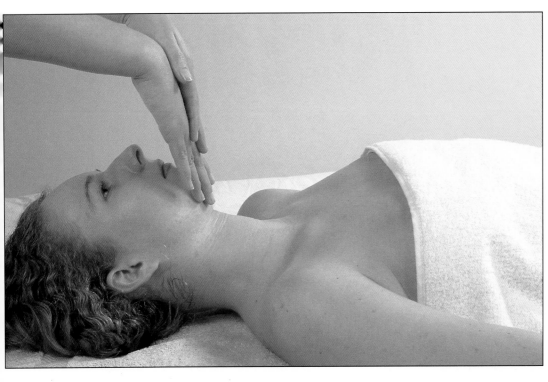

4 Repeat once again, but this time finish by bringing both hands up to the jawline with the fingers resting lightly under the centre of the jaw.

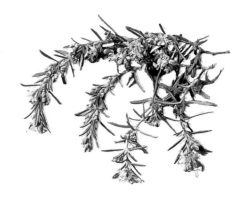

Use rosemary oil to help strengthen the mind in times of mental fatigue and emotional stress.

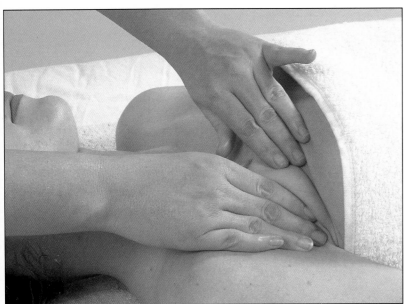

5 With both hands, knead the fleshy area in front of the armpit. Pick up and release the muscles, squeezing them from one hand to the other.

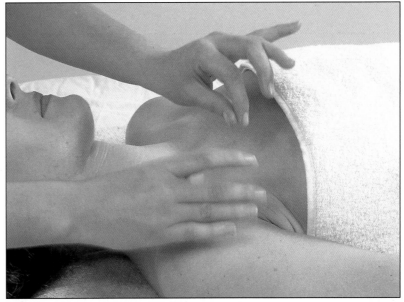

6 On the same fleshy area, lightly pinch the surface muscles between the thumb and first finger. Alternate the hands swiftly in a rhythmical action, checking with your partner that this causes no discomfort. Repeat steps 2 and 3 to soothe the area you have worked on, then repeat the whole sequence on the left side of the chest.

THE SHOULDERS AND NECK

Tension in the chest can exacerbate inflexibility and stiffness in the neck and shoulders. We tend to raise the shoulders towards the ears, until they become set rigid with tension.

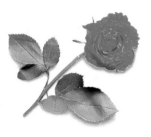

The uplifting properties of rose oil can help ease strain in the neck caused by nervous tension.

1 Place both hands fairly firmly, side by side, over the front of the chest.

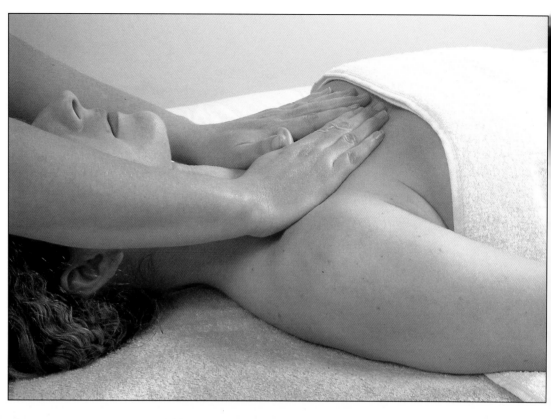

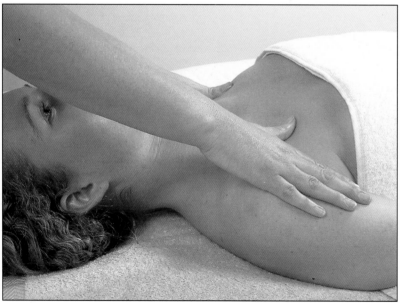

2 Sweep them out towards each shoulder with firm effleurage strokes, taking them over the shoulders, around under the upper back and up the back of the neck.

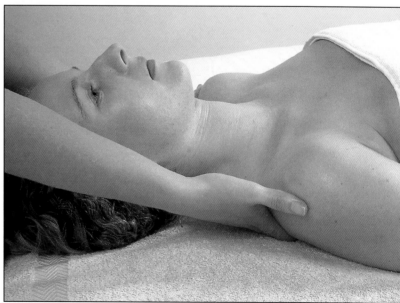

3 When you take the movement around the back and the neck, gently lift the weight of your partner to give the muscles a gentle stretch.

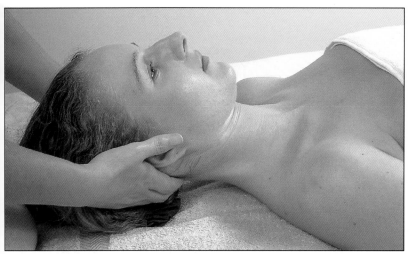

4 With your fingertips, work with circular pressures up the back of the neck to the base of the skull. These should be small, firm rotations, which you can feel easing taut muscles. You should spend some time on this area, which is often extremely tense; take the trouble to release as much tension as possible.

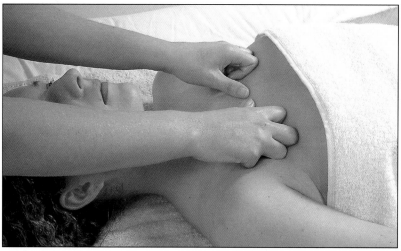

5 With loose fists, use the knuckle area to ripple your fingers in semicircular frictions all over the upper chest. Keep the half circles fairly small and apply firm pressure on the fleshier area, but avoid working directly on the collarbone.

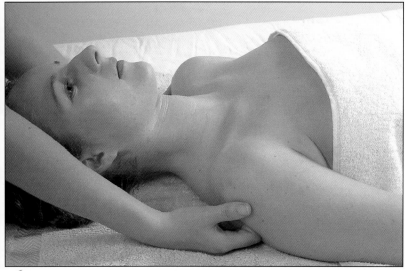

6 Bring your loose fists under the upper back and continue to knead behind the shoulders and around the base of the neck.

7 Finish with several effleurage strokes, starting at the front of the chest and stroking the hands over each shoulder and up behind the neck.

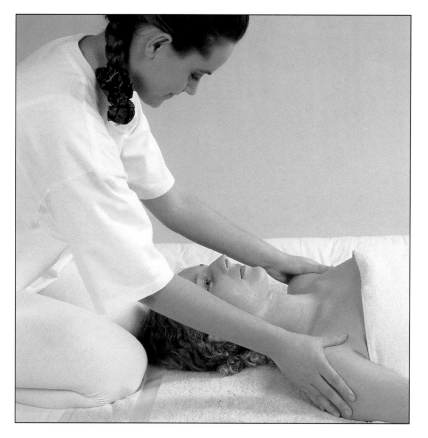

THE FACE

The face constantly mirrors our health and emotions. Stress and tension are reflected in a furrowed brow, and lines around the eyes, mouth and jawline. A facial massage can soothe away headaches, anxiety and exhaustion and replace them with a feeling of serenity. It improves the circulation, giving the skin a healthy glow.

If your partner wears contact lenses, make sure they are removed before you start a face massage. Use a little light oil, and don't let it get too near or go in the eyes, mouth or nose. Make sure the hair is held securely away from the face and neck in a soft hairband. Keep the hands relaxed. You may be surprised to find that the face is less fragile than it looks and you can apply quite deep pressure without causing discomfort.

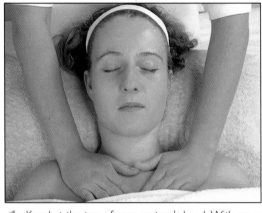

1 Kneel at the top of your partner's head. With your hands placed over the collarbone, pointing away from you, begin with some gentle effleurage strokes.

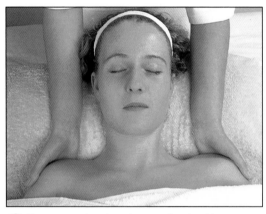

2 Sweep your hands out across the shoulders, keeping the pressure light.

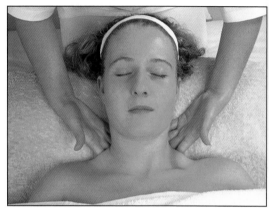

3 In a continuous movement, bring your hands up around the back of the neck to the nape; pause for a moment, increasing the pressure slightly with the fingertips, then release and lift your hands away. Repeat this effleurage sequence at least three times.

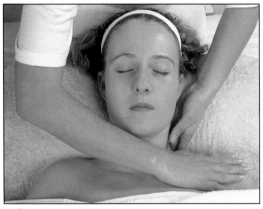

4 Bring your right arm across the front of your partner so that the hand supports the left shoulder. Using light upward strokes, sweep your left hand up from the top of the shoulder, up the side of the neck to the edge of the jaw. Repeat three times.

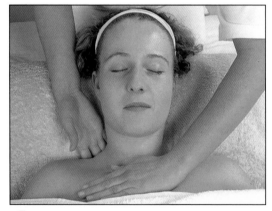

5 Now repeat this movement on the other side of the neck.

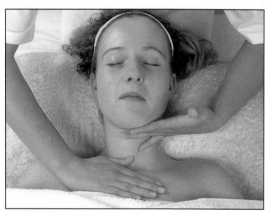

6 Starting with both hands over the front of the chest, fingers pointing toward each other, lightly sweep the flat of one hand up the front of the neck to the jaw, flicking the hand away when you get there. As you flick the first hand away, bring the second up, so that you stroke with alternate hands. Repeat this stroking and flicking movement several times.

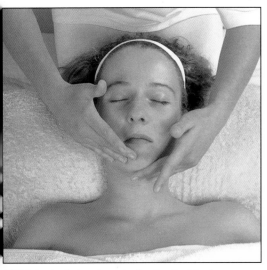

7 Bring both hands up to the front of the jaw. Alternately sweep one hand and then the other up along the jawline towards the ear. Repeat the movement several times.

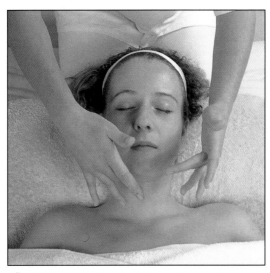

8 Briskly tap the length of the jawline using the middle and ring fingers, starting from the centre front and working towards the ears. This should have a stimulating effect, so keep the patting movement quick and fairly firm.

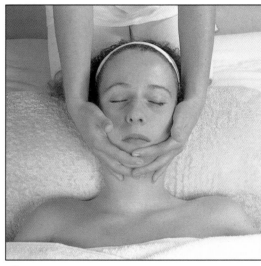

9 Afterwards, soothe the area by cradling the face gently with both hands. Pause for several moments, then release the hands.

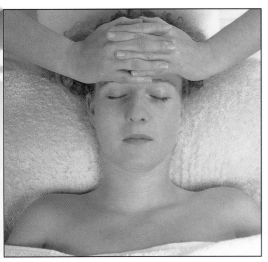

10 Bring your hands up to the forehead. Loosely interlock your fingers, and using the palms, apply gentle pressure over the forehead. Slowly unlock the fingers to release. Repeat three times.

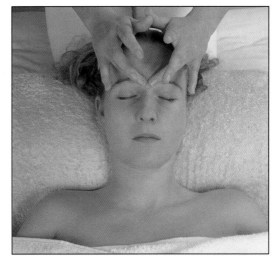

11 Starting with the third finger of each hand placed on the bridge of the nose, stroke out over the brows towards the temples at each side of the forehead. Come up the forehead a little and, starting again with both fingers at the centre front, repeat the strokes out towards the hairline. Repeat a couple of times more, bringing the fingers higher up the forehead each time, until the whole forehead is covered.

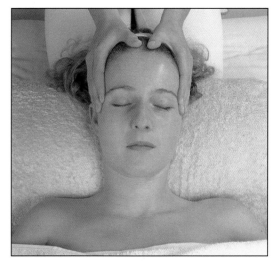

12 To finish, place your hands on each side of your partner's head, and pause for a few seconds before lifting them away.

THE ABDOMEN

Many people feel exposed and vulnerable when baring their abdomen, so you will need to be particularly sensitive to your partner when it comes to this part of the massage. Start with very gentle strokes, but try to be confident, as a gentle touch which is also tentative can feel unnerving for your partner.

Massage of the abdomen calms the nerves and can soothe stomach aches if they are caused by tension, poor digestion or period pains. It also stimulates the digestive organs so that elimination is improved. You should wait for at least an hour after your partner's meal before giving an abdominal massage.

Rhythm

It helps to start and finish the massage by focusing on your partner's breathing, so that your strokes coincide with their body's natural rhythm. To begin, try slowly stroking your hands up from the lower abdomen to the chest on inhalation, and down the sides of the body on exhalation.

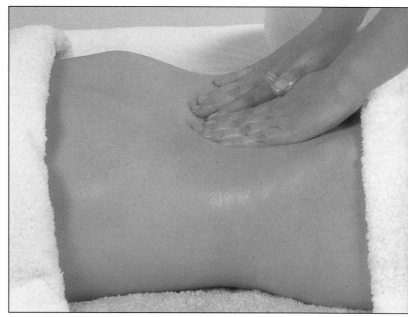

1 Kneel beside your partner at hip level. Make contact by gently placing your hands together in a diamond shape over the lower abdomen, pointing towards the head. Keep the fingers together and the hands relaxed. Ask your partner to breathe into the abdomen so you can feel it expand and contract. Work with the breath.

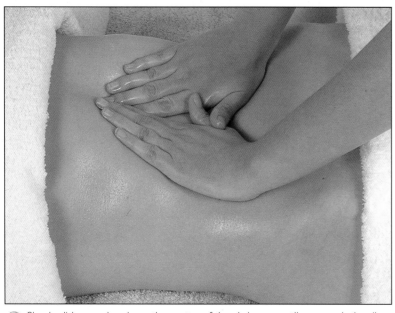

2 Slowly slide your hands up the centre of the abdomen until you reach the ribs, making sure the pressure is even and not too firm.

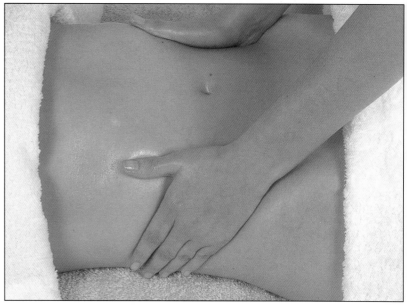

3 Continue the movement by sweeping the hands out and around the sides of the waist. As you take them out from the ribs towards the sides, you can apply a little more pressure, so that you feel the muscles being drawn outward.

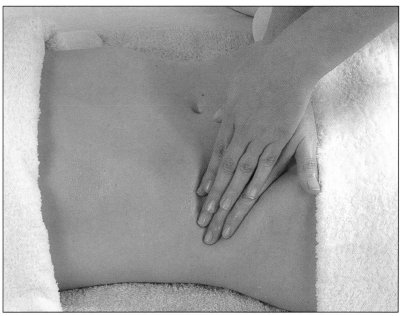

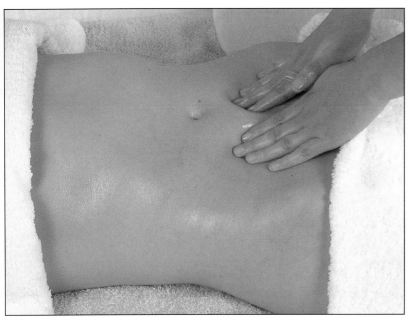

4 Return to the starting position, with both hands placed on the lower abdomen, and repeat this continuous movement several times.

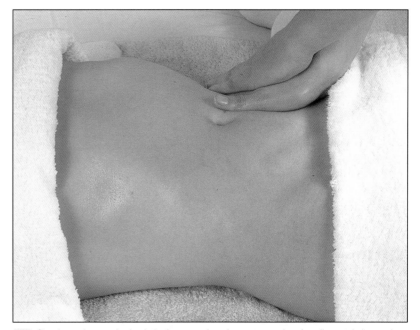

5 Place both hands on the right-hand side of your partner's lower abdomen, ready to circle the navel. Rest your left hand over the right for support.

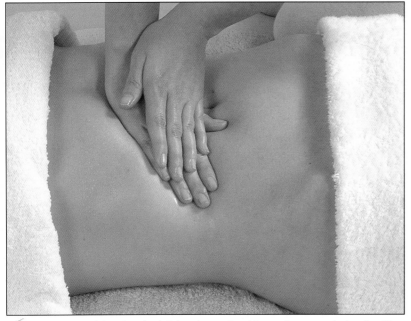

6 Stroke upward, keeping the left hand over the right, until you reach the ribs. The pressure can be quite firm to stimulate the digestive system. Keep the stroke smooth and continuous.

7 Continue the stroke by bringing your hands across under the ribs, and down the left side of your partner's abdomen. Repeat the navel-circling movement three times, each time returning to the centre of the lower abdomen, and always working up the right side, across and down the left side.

THE WAIST

Your movements around the waist area should be firm and stimulating, but lighten your touch as your hands cross the abdomen to reach the opposite side of the body.

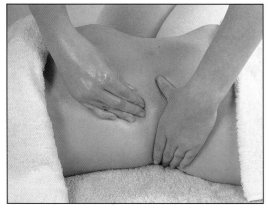

1 To begin the massage, knead around the waist area by squeezing and releasing the flesh from one hand to the other.

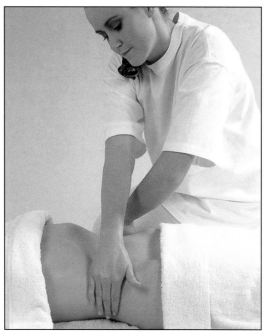

2 Cross your hands over your partner's waist so the palms are grasping each side of the midriff. Briskly draw them up the sides of the waist, uncrossing them as they meet and turning the palms to travel down the other side. Draw up again and recross the hands to reach your starting position. Repeat four times.

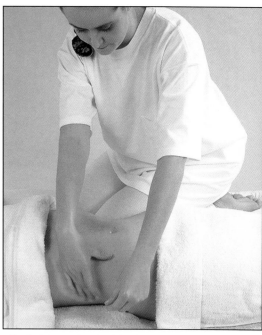

3 Starting at the far side of the waist, lightly pinch the flesh between fingers and thumbs with brisk, short movements. Repeat the same movement on the other side of the waist.

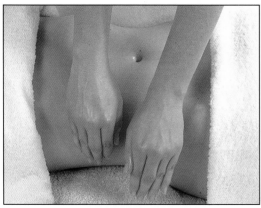

4 Lightly cup the side of the waist, keeping the pace fast and stimulating, but at the same time checking that it is not causing discomfort. The action should not be painful, but should be enough to increase the flow of blood to the area.

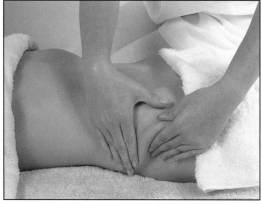

5 Working on the top of the hip area, squeeze and release the flesh in a kneading movement, using deep and stimulating pressure.

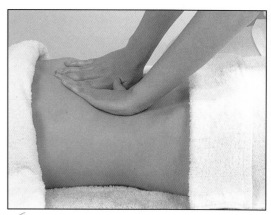

6 Finish the massage of the abdomen by repeating the soothing effleurage strokes from the beginning of the previous sequence. End with both hands placed over the centre of the abdomen, fingers pointing towards the head. Hold for a few seconds before lifting your hands off.

THE BACK OF THE BODY

Ask your partner to turn over on to their front, ready for you to start work on the back of the legs and buttocks.

THE LEGS

Effleurage on the legs can stimulate other body functions and can help improve their efficiency. Poor circulation and a sluggish lymphatic system can be considerably improved by a good leg massage. Tiredness and heaviness in the legs is alleviated and your partner should be left with a feeling of renewed energy.

Complete the whole back of leg massage on one leg before moving around to the other side of your partner to repeat the sequence. Cover the leg you have worked on with a towel to keep the muscles warm.

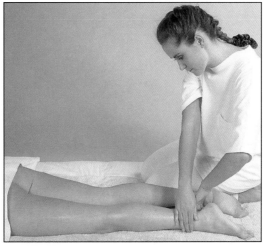

1 Start by kneeling at one side of your partner's ankles. You should be able to work on both legs from the same side quite easily. Begin by working on the leg furthest away from you and cross your hands over the back of the ankle.

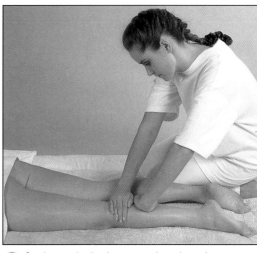

2 Stroke up the leg in a smooth and continuous movement, with the right hand leading the left. When you reach the back of the knee, pause for two or three seconds.

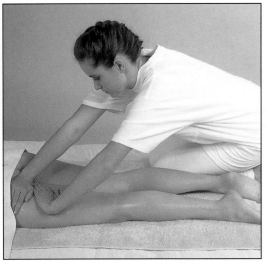

3 Carry the stroke up the leg and cross the hands at the top of the thigh, keeping the pressure even and light throughout the movement.

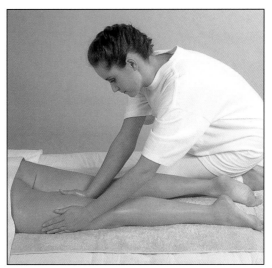

4 Bring your hands back down the sides of the leg to the ankle. Repeat the sequence three times, each time increasing the pressure slightly.

CAUTION: You will need to take certain precautions if your partner has varicose veins. Never knead or put any pressure on varicose veins, and only massage the part of the leg higher than the area with the vein (that is, only massage closer to the heart); never massage on or below the vein.

THE UPPER LEGS AND BUTTOCKS

The backs of the legs and buttocks offer plenty of scope for massage techniques. Most people can take plenty of firm massage on the larger muscles in the thighs and buttocks. The fleshy parts are ideal for kneading and squeezing, and firm pressure can feel wonderfully satisfying. Kneel at your partner's side and work on the leg opposite.

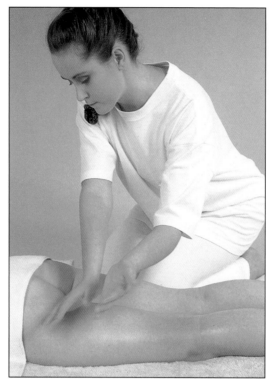

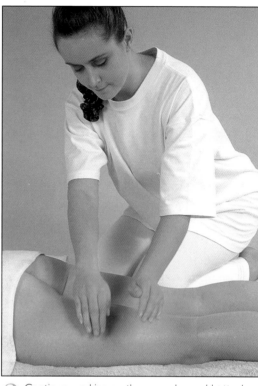

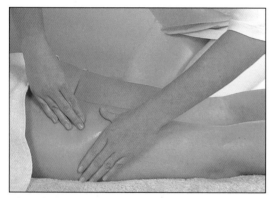

1 Using a firm kneading movement, squeeze and release the back of the thigh muscles, working up to the buttock. You should be able to pick up quite a large area of muscle between the hands.

2 With the outside edge of the hands, do some short, sharp hacking movements. Alternate the hands in a quick, repetitive action. Continue the hacking all over the back of the upper leg and the buttock.

3 Continue working on the upper leg and buttock, with some cupping. The cupping action should be short and fast to stimulate the whole area.

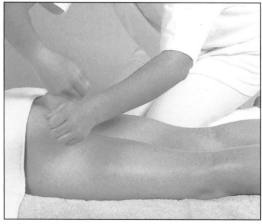

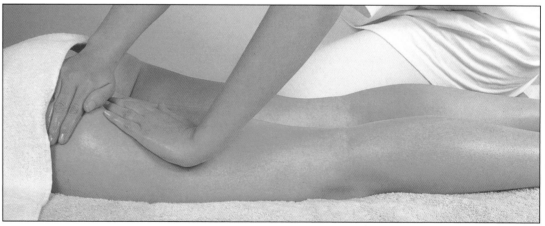

4 With loose fists, briskly pound the top and outside of the thigh. You can use the backs of your fingers or the outside edge of the fists. Use a firmer knuckling action over the buttock area.

5 Follow this sequence of friction movements with soothing effleurage strokes from the back of the knee to the top of the thigh, sweeping out and back down the leg to the knee.

THE CALVES

Move down to kneel beside your partner's ankles, and work on the calf of the same leg, lightly oiling your hands again if necessary.

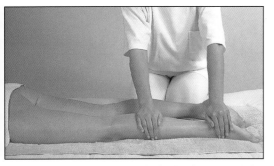

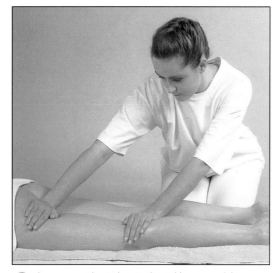

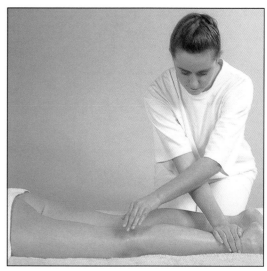

1 Start with both hands on the back of your partner's ankle. Smooth your right hand up towards the knee, keeping your left hand on the ankle for support. Keep the pressure light on the back of the knee.

2 As you continue the stroke, taking your right hand up towards the top of the thigh, slide your left hand up the lower leg to the back of the knee. Try to do this in one single, flowing movement.

3 Without pausing, bring your right hand in one stroke back down the leg. Slide the left hand off the knee, so the right hand can continue down to the ankle. Repeat the effleurage stroke at least three times.

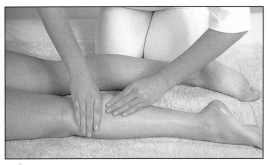

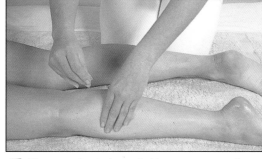

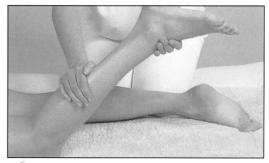

4 Knead the calf with both hands, working from the ankle up to the knee, but do not knead the back of the knee. If the muscles are tight, this action may feel uncomfortable, so do ask if the pressure is right.

5 Do some short, sharp pinching movements all over the calf muscle, again checking that you are not hurting your partner.

6 Supporting your partner's leg in the left hand, slide your right hand up from the back of the ankle to the knee. Keep the pressure as firm as is comfortable. Repeat three times before gently lowering the leg.

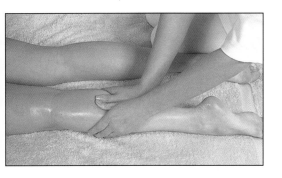

7 With your thumbs together, start at the back of the ankle and work up the back of the calf to the knee, applying pressure firm enough to release tightness in these muscles. When you reach the back of the knee, lighten the pressure and sweep your hands back down the sides of the leg to the ankle. Repeat three times, then repeat the effleurage strokes from the beginning of the whole sequence to soothe the leg.

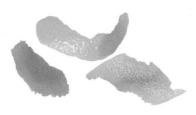

Orange essential oil is known to act as an antidote to water retention in the lower legs.

THE BACK AND SHOULDERS

The back is an area of great strength and mobility, and it is the main supportive structure of the body. It therefore warrants more attention than most other areas. By working on the back, you can reach nerves affecting every part of the body.

Full back massage, with emphasis on the spine and lower back, greatly alleviates the effects of stress throughout the body, enhancing physical and psychological well-being. Smooth, flowing strokes stretch the muscles and tissues around the contours of the back, and help to restore flexibility for health and mobility, while stronger strokes along the spinal muscles and over the lower back bring deeper relief to aching or knotted muscles.

With your initial effleurage strokes, concentrate on finding areas of tension and tightness.

1 Before you begin to work on the back, make sure your partner is comfortable, lying face down with arms resting beside the face. Support the forehead with a rolled towel, and if it is helpful use a pillow or rolled towel under the chest. It is a good idea to have the hair clear of the back of the neck, secured in a soft band. Kneel beside your partner's hip.

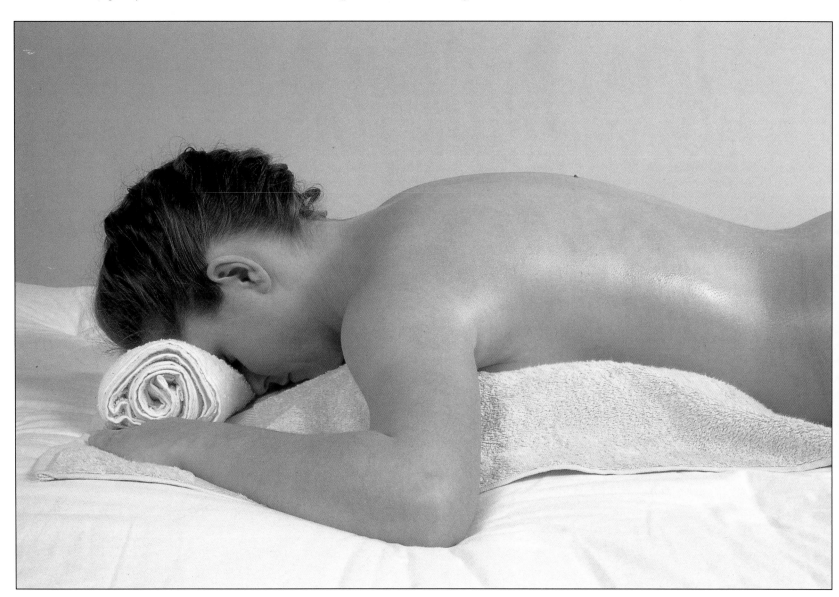

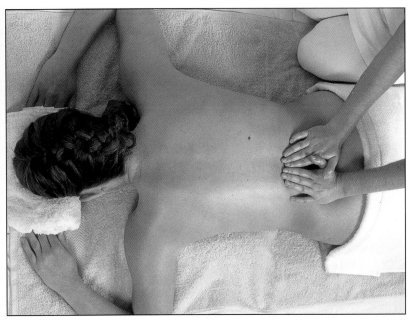

2 Starting at the lower back, begin the effleurage strokes. With thumbs crossed to connect the hands together, move slowly up the centre of the back, putting firm pressure on the fingertips.

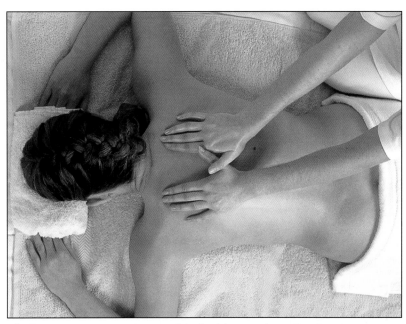

3 Take the stroke up to the top of the back in a continuous movement.

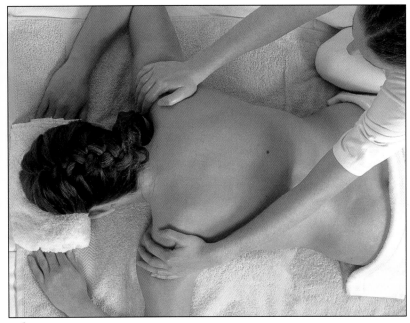

4 Without a pause, separate the hands at the top of the back, sweeping them out and around the shoulders.

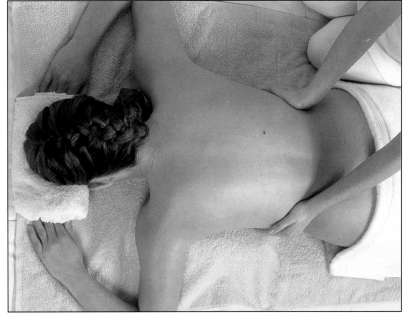

5 Continue the stroke, bringing both hands down the sides to the lower back, ready to begin again. Repeat this effleurage sequence three times, oiling your hands each time.

THE SHOULDERS

Work through this sequence from your original position, then move to the other side of your partner and repeat the steps on the other shoulder.

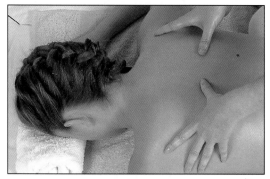

1 Using your thumbs on each side of the spine, start level with the shoulder blades and make circling pressure movements. Work quite firmly into the muscles, but remember to ask your partner if the movement is causing them any discomfort.

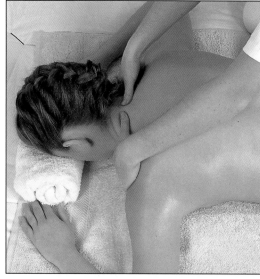

2 Continue working up each side of the spine until you reach the nape of the neck. Keep the amount of pressure even, and try to maintain a steady rhythm for the stroke.

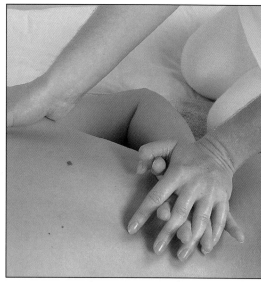

3 Carefully bring your partner's right arm across the hollow of the back and clasp the hand with your left hand. The shoulder blade should now stick out slightly. With your right thumb, make circular pressure movements over the shoulder area. Strong muscles support the shoulder blade and you can work firmly under the bone to release tightness here.

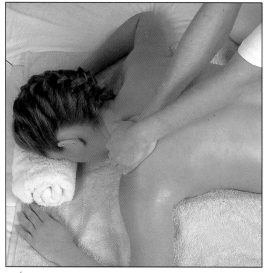

4 Having replaced your partner's arm, work in small circular movements from the base of the neck out over the shoulder. Rest your left hand over your right to increase the pressure.

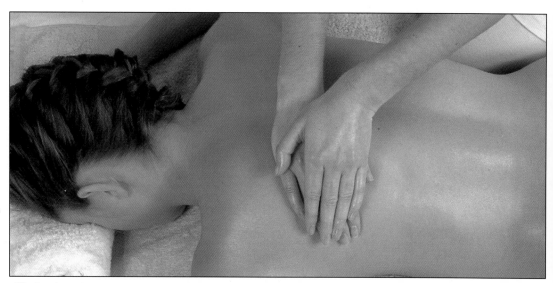

5 Continue the movement around to the shoulder blade, using firm pressure to release tension in the muscle. Repeat steps 1–5 on the other side of your partner's body.

THE BACK

Avoid using percussion strokes such as hacking and cupping on the kidneys, which are level with the waistline in the centre of the back.

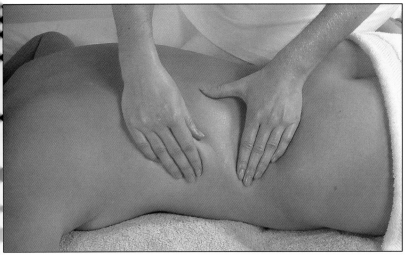

1 Knead the far side of the back firmly with both hands, beginning at the outer side of the waist. Pick up, roll and release the muscles, alternately pressing one hand towards the other. Continue kneading up the back until you reach the shoulders. Start again at the waist but this time come closer to the spine and repeat the line of kneading up the back. Repeat on the near side of the back – you should be able to do this without altering your position.

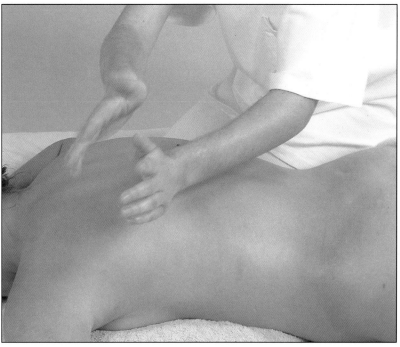

2 Using the outer edges of your hands, briskly and rhythmically hack from the lower back up to the shoulders, but avoid the bony shoulder blade. Try to visualize each side of the back divided into three sections so that you cover the whole back thoroughly.

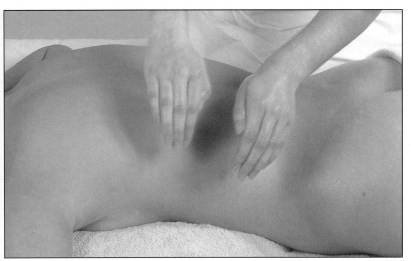

3 Start cupping from the lower back, working upward and across the shoulders. The action should be quick, with alternate hands striking the back briskly.

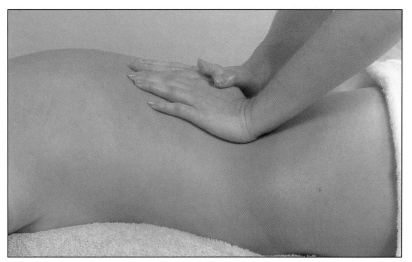

4 Repeat the effleurage strokes from the beginning of the back massage sequence to soothe the back. Repeat several times.

THE SPINE

It is important to remember never to massage directly on the spine itself, although working down each side of the spine can be highly beneficial.

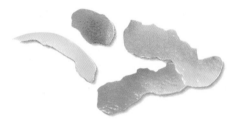

Lemon oil can refresh and clarify thought. Use it on the back for a thoroughly uplifting massage.

1 With loose fists, and thumbs crossed for support, push the top of the hands up each side of the spine to the nape of the neck.

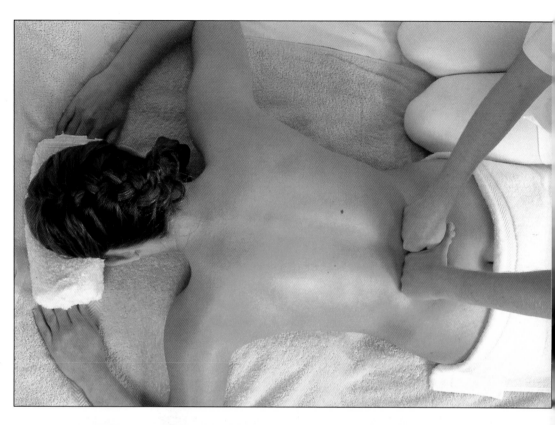

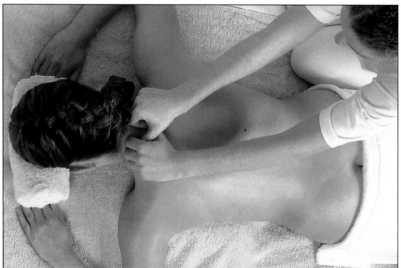

2 Uncurl the fingers when you reach the nape and sweep them back down the sides of the back. Repeat these strokes three times.

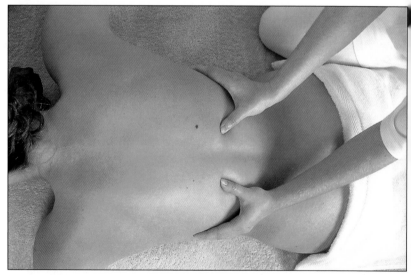

3 Starting at the lower back, place the thumbs on either side of the spine, resting your hands at either side of the back. Rotate the thumbs in small circles, travelling up the sides of the spine until you reach the hairline. Use firm pressure. Reverse the movement, circling your thumbs back down each side of the spine.

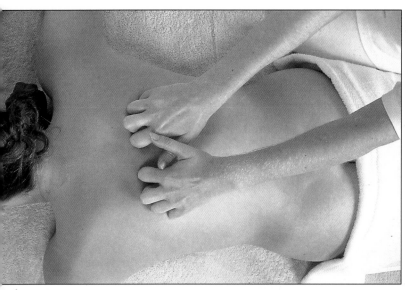

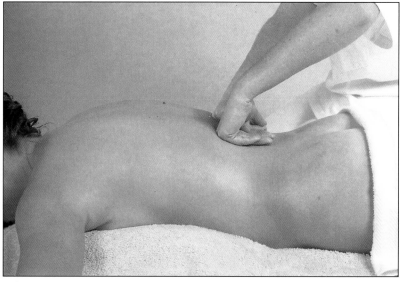

4 Starting at the lower back, use loose knuckles, crossing your thumbs over each other for support, to work up either side of the spine and back down again. Repeat twice.

5 Using the backs of your hands and starting at the lower back, push up either side of the spine to just above the waistline. Then sweep your hands outward and back down around the hips. Repeat three times.

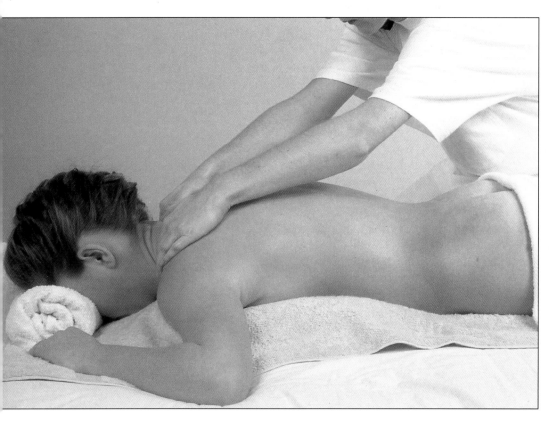

6 To finish the massage, repeat the effleurage strokes from the beginning of the sequence, starting at the lower back and working up the back, around the shoulders and down again to the lower back, in a continuous sweeping movement.

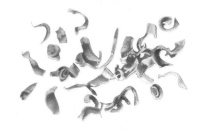

A full back massage using oil of neroli will soothe anxiety and encourage a sense of peace.

Instant Massage

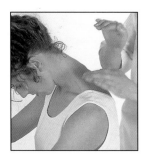

Do you come home at the end of the day with your neck and shoulders feeling as if they were set in concrete? Does stress leave your back stiff and aching? Anyone who experiences the physical tensions that accompany stressful situations will find that massage is one of the most successful ways to relax painful, knotted muscles. Most of us almost unconsciously rub tense, aching spots to obtain some instant relief; correctly performed, massage can have a wonderful effect on tense muscles and on our whole sense of well-being, even if you only have a few minutes.

One of the great advantages of massage is that it can be adapted to virtually any situation. You can relax most completely if you have a partner to massage you, but it is almost as effective if you do it on yourself. Some of the strokes are versatile enough to apply not only at home but also in the workplace or even on a bus, since it is not essential for you to be naked or even partially clothed for your tired, aching muscles to be massaged. Massage through clothes can be very effective, though a little more pressure may need to be applied. You can apply a particular sequence of strokes to ease specific muscular aches or, if you have a little more time, combine several of the sequences that follow for a relaxing but quick and easy massage, any time, anywhere.

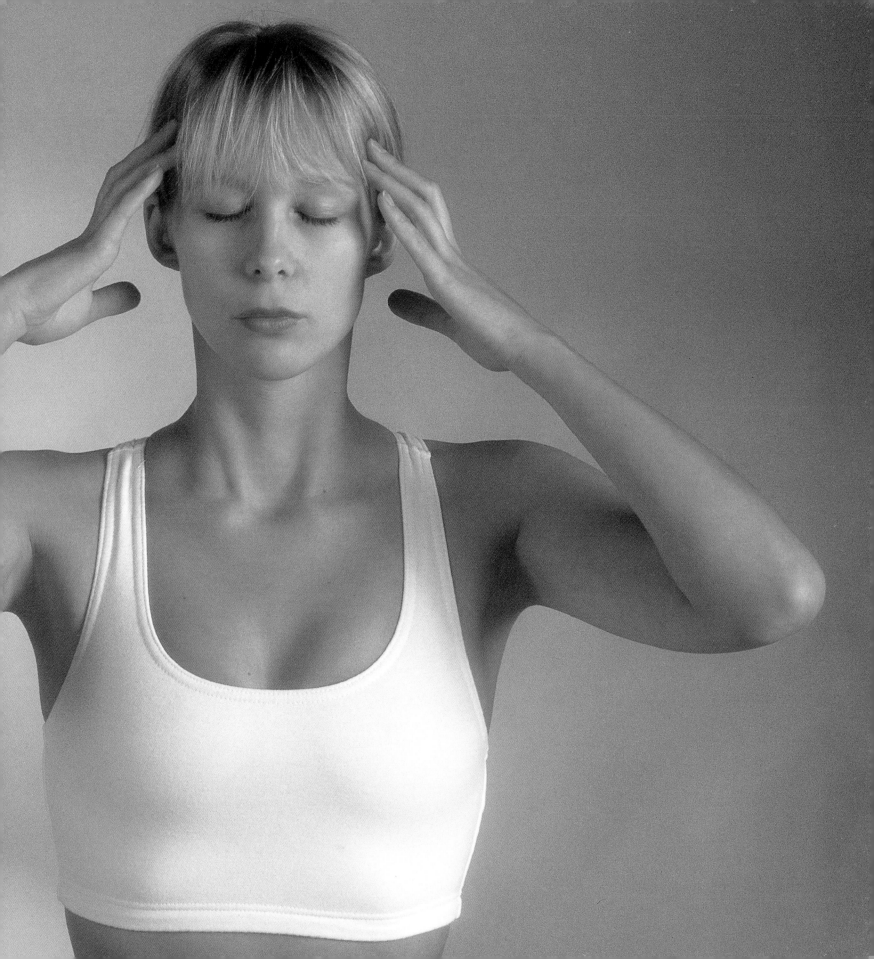

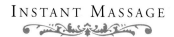

10-MINUTE MASSAGE

Sometimes the idea of having the tension in your shoulders and neck instantly massaged away is particularly tempting. Without stopping to find the right place and time to undress, a shoulder massage can be done with the minimum of disruption. There are times when the best therapy you can give your partner is a quick shoulder and back massage while sitting comfortably on an upright chair. It can be done through light clothing if that is simpler, and there is no need to use oil if you prefer not to.

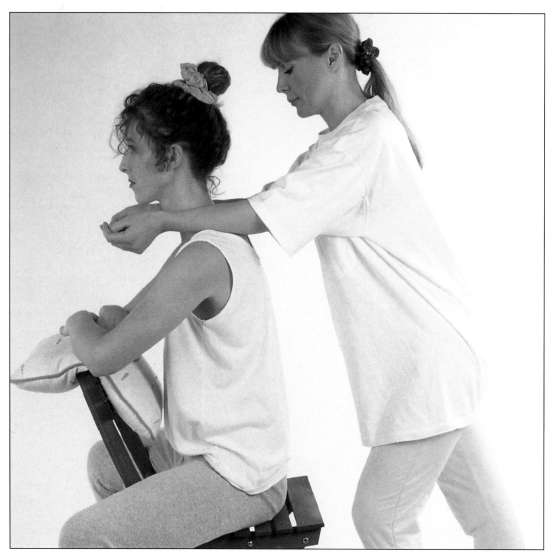

1 Ask your partner to sit astride a chair, facing the back. You can offer a folded towel or cushion for comfort. Standing behind your partner, begin by leaning on your forearms so that your weight presses down gently on to the fleshy part of the shoulders.

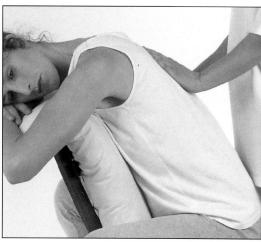

2 With your partner leaning forward, use effleurage strokes from the bottom of the shoulder blades, up the back and out over the tops of the shoulders, to finish at the tops of the arms. Repeat four times.

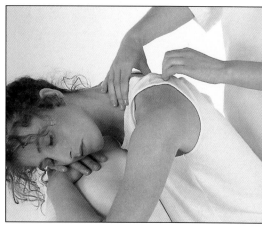

3 With a firm petrissage, use both hands to knead out along the shoulders from the sides of the neck to the upper arms.

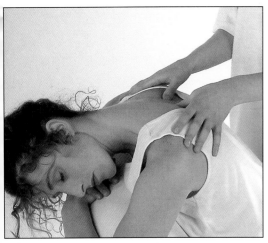

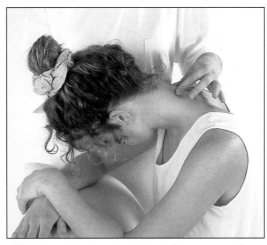

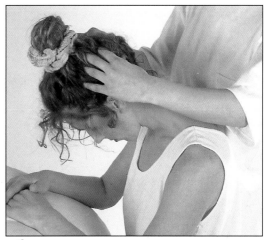

4 Starting as far down the lower back as you can, work up the spine with small circular friction strokes. Continue up the sides of the neck to the base of the skull, then glide back down and work up again, this time moving out over the shoulders as you reach the top of the back.

5 Move around to the side and tilt your partner's head forward, supporting it with one hand. With the thumb and finger of the other hand, grasp the neck firmly and massage with circular movements, working up the neck and into the base of the skull.

6 Working from behind your partner again, massage the back of the head with both hands, coming over the forehead and down to the temples with small circular pressures, moving the scalp against the skull. Lighten your touch at the temples.

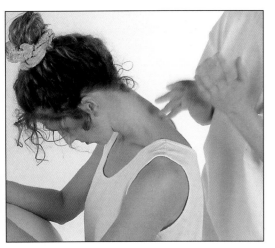

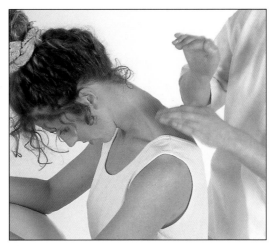

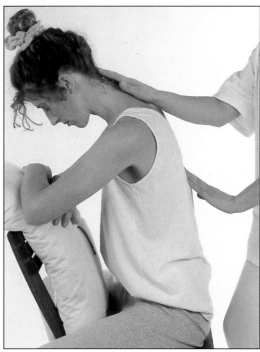

7 First on one side, and then on the other, do some hacking across the fleshy parts of the shoulders and upper back, using the outer side of your hands to make short, brisk movements. Keep your wrists and hands very relaxed.

8 Continue with a brisk cupping action across each shoulder, working on one side at a time. Remember to keep your wrists and hands relaxed as you work.

9 Finish the sequence by gently stroking down the entire back with one hand following the other. Repeat five times, with each stroke lighter than the last.

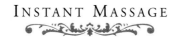

INSTANT SELF-MASSAGE

Self-massage is a quick and effective way to relieve tension or pick yourself up at any time of day, whether you need to relieve a particular group of tired, aching muscles, or to re-energize yourself when you have run out of steam.

SIMPLE REVITALIZER

At any time during a busy day your energy can flag. If you need to be bright and alert for a meeting, a long drive, picking up the kids or going to a party, give yourself an instant "waker-upper" with this short routine.

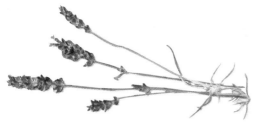

The balancing effect of lavender oil makes it a wonderful stress-beater.

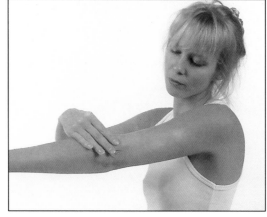

1 Use a fast kneading action on the arms, working rapidly from the wrist to the shoulder and back again with a firm squeezing movement, to invigorate the arm and shoulder.

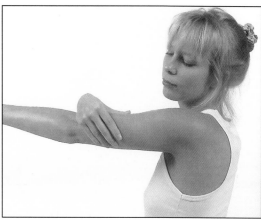

2 Rub swiftly up the outside of the arm to stimulate the circulation. Repeat several times, working in an upwards direction each time, to encourage blood flow back to the heart. Repeat the sequence on the other arm and shoulder.

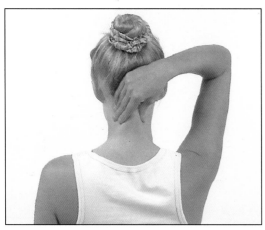

3 With the fingers and thumb of one hand, firmly squeeze the neck muscles using a circular motion.

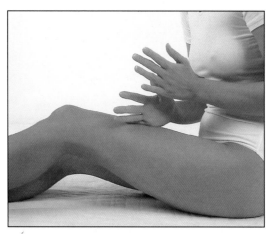

4 With the outside edges of the hands, lightly hack along the front of the thighs, using a rapid motion. The hands should spring up from the muscles.

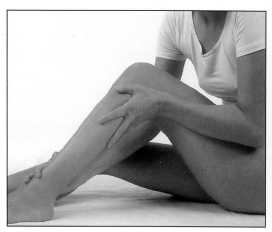

5 Rub the calves vigorously to loosen the muscles and to get the blood moving. If possible, do this with the legs bent. Make each stroke from the ankle to the knee, using alternate hands. Finally, stand up and shake your whole body, to let go of any remaining stiffness and tension.

HEAD REVITALIZER

Headaches can have a multitude of causes, such as spending too much time in front of a VDU, anxiety, insomnia, fatigue or sinus congestion. However, the most common cause is tension arising from periods of stress. Use this self-massage sequence to help ease a headache, whatever its cause. You can also use it at any time to increase your vitality and help you to focus your mind.

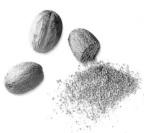

Nutmeg essential oil has a warming, stimulating effect, and can help relieve nervous fatigue.

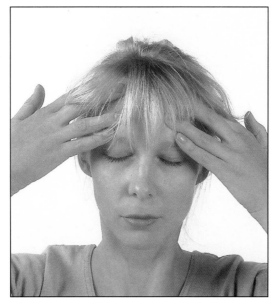

1 Use small, circling movements with the fingers, working steadily from the forehead down around the temples and over the cheeks.

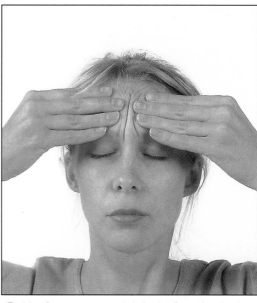

2 Use firm pressure and circle the fingertips slowly to ease tension out of all the facial muscles.

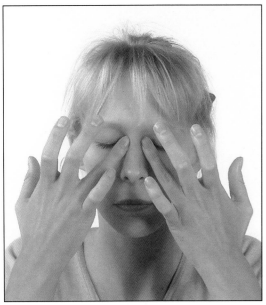

3 Press gently around the eye socket, by the nose, using the third finger of each hand.

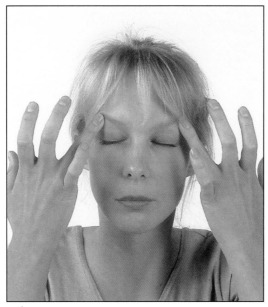

4 Smooth firmly around the arc of your eye socket beneath your brow bone.

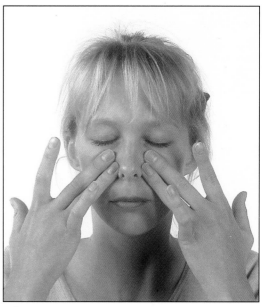

5 Work across the cheeks and along each side of the nose, then move out to the jawline where a lot of tension is held. Try not to pull downwards on the skin – let the circling movements help to smooth the stress away and gently lift the face as you work.

TENSE NECK EASER

As you get tired, your posture tends to droop, making your neck and shoulders ache. Practise these movements and help release any mounting tension in these areas before your shoulders become permanently hunched up.

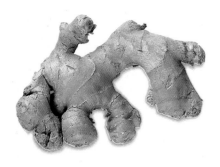

Ginger oil will help counteract all manner of aches and pains.

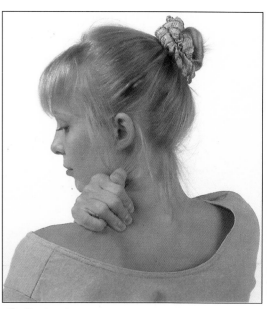

1 A simple movement is to shrug your shoulders, exaggerating their contraction by lifting them up as far as possible and then letting them drop down and relax completely.

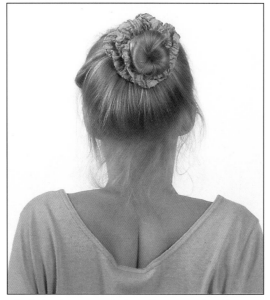

2 Firmly grip your opposite shoulder with your hand and use a squeezing motion to loosen the tension in the muscles. If your working arm starts to ache, rest for a moment before continuing.

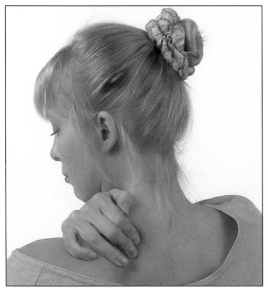

3 Move slowly along the shoulder, squeezing the flesh firmly several times between your fingers and the ball of your hand. Repeat on the opposite side, using the other hand.

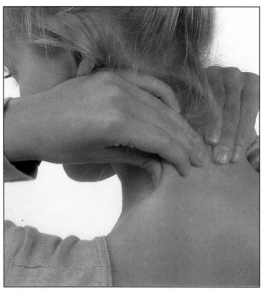

4 With the fingers and thumbs of both hands, grip the back of the neck and squeeze in a circular motion to help relax the muscles leading up either side of the neck. Work up to the base of the skull and down again to the shoulders.

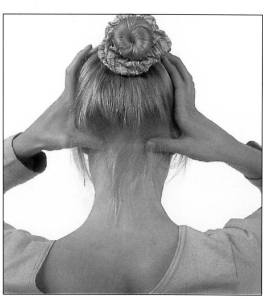

5 To work more deeply into the neck, move the thumbs in a circular movement across the neck and right up into the base of the skull. You will feel the bone as you apply moderate pressure.

TONIC FOR ACHING LEGS

Any occupation that involves long periods of standing still can create real problems for circulation in the legs, leading to tired, aching limbs, swollen ankles or cramp. It is, of course, essential to try to move around as much as possible, but a quick self-massage at the end of the day can help considerably in reducing stiffness and sluggish blood flow in the legs. Remember to take extreme care if your partner suffers from varicose veins. Do not apply pressure to the vein itself, and massage only on the part of the leg above the vein (that is, nearer to the heart); never work below the vein.

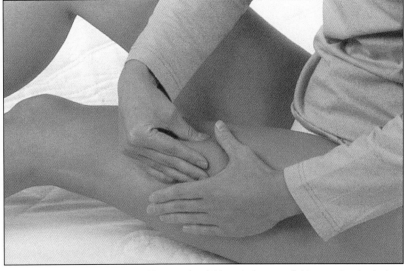

1 Start a leg massage by working on the thighs, so that any fluid retention in the calves will have somewhere to go as the upper leg relaxes. Knead the flesh of the thigh between the fingers and thumb, squeezing with each hand alternately and working from the knee to the hip and back. Repeat on the other thigh.

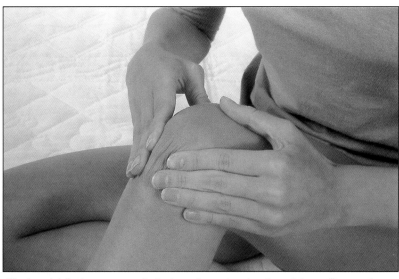

2 Around the knees, use a similar kneading action, but for a lighter effect use just the fingers and work in smaller circles.

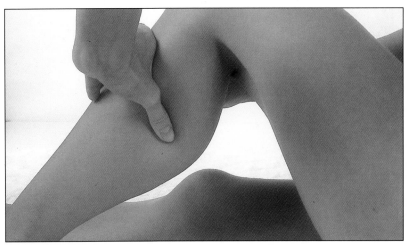

3 Bend your leg, and if possible raise the foot on a chair or handy ledge. With your thumbs, work on the back of each calf with a circular, kneading action. Repeat a few times, each time working from the ankle up the leg to the knee.

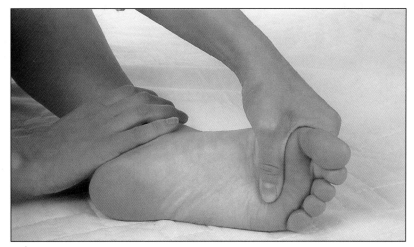

4 Squeeze the foot, loosening up the muscles and gently stretching the arch. Use firm pressure with your thumb to stretch the foot. Repeat on the other foot.

CHEST AND ABDOMEN RELEASER

The front of your body is an area where emotional tension is often stored; bottling up your feelings can create tight muscles across your chest or in your abdomen. Massage treatments on these areas often trigger the release of deep-seated emotions, and need a skilled, sensitive approach. Self-massage is, however, very helpful, both in easing tense muscles and in helping to recognize where stored tensions lie. An awareness of the effects of stress is the first step towards letting go of it.

1 Using the thumb and fingers, take a good grip of the pectoral muscles leading from the chest to the shoulder, and knead them firmly.

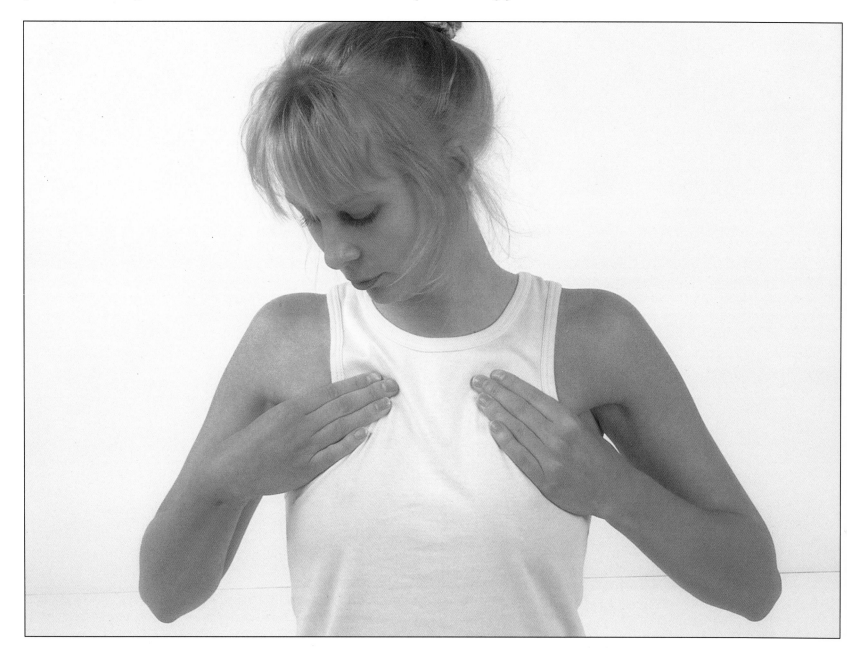

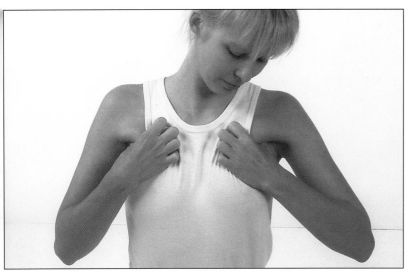

2 Be careful if you have any tenderness in the lymph glands under the armpits. Women should also go gently if they have tender, swollen breasts; for example when pre-menstrual.

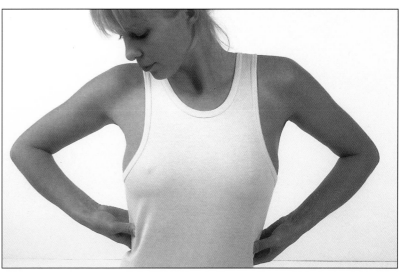

3 Using a couple of fingers, feel in between the ribs for the intercostal muscles, and work firmly along between each rib, moving the fingers in tiny circles, repeating on each side.

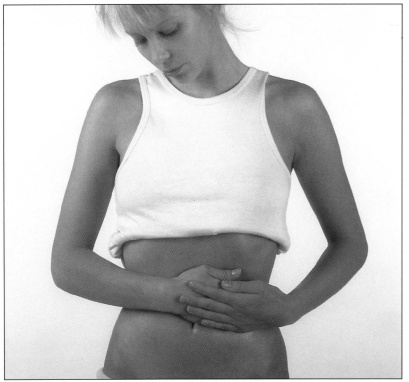

4 Place your hands on your abdomen, and, pressing gently, work around slowly in a clockwise direction.

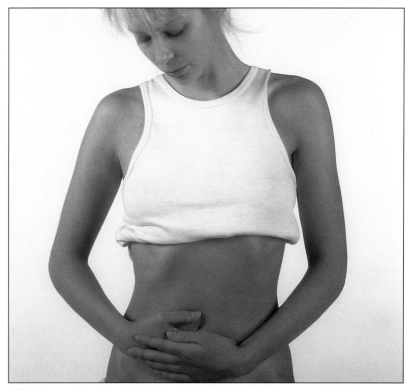

5 If it is comfortable, repeat twice with increasing pressure; ease off if this becomes painful. Working in this direction encourages digestive and bowel action.

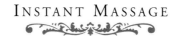

OFFICE MASSAGE

Massage is a highly versatile skill, and can be applied in many situations. When one of your work colleagues complains of tense, aching shoulders or back, you can do something about it. This five-minute sequence can be done at a desk, and can be wonderfully effective in refreshing and re-energizing people.

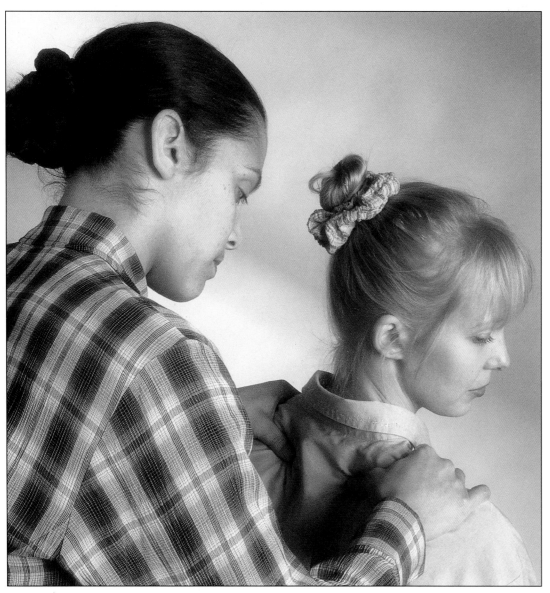

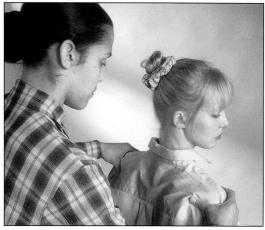

2 Knead both shoulders at the same time, with a firm squeezing movement; adjust the pressure you use according to the amount of clothing and the degree of discomfort your partner is experiencing.

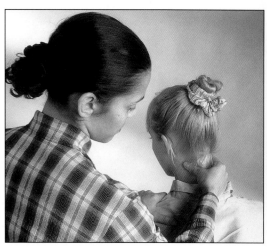

3 Using your fingers, knead in small circles up and down the back of the neck. Always try to support the head with your free hand while you are working on the neck.

1 Standing behind your seated colleague, place your hands on both their shoulders, with your thumbs towards you and your fingers to the front.

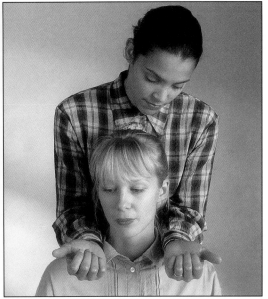

4 Place your forearms over the shoulders and press down with your body weight to squeeze and stretch the trapezius muscles.

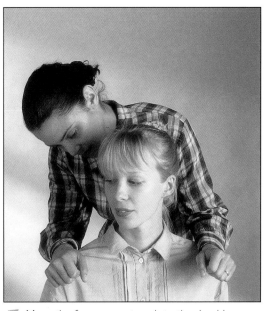

5 Move the forearms outwards to the shoulders, maintaining a firm pressure all the time.

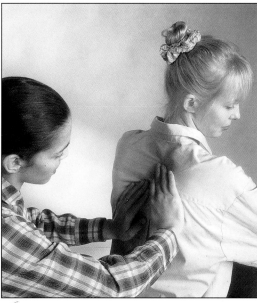

6 Using your fingers, make firm circling motions down the back, to either side of the spine.

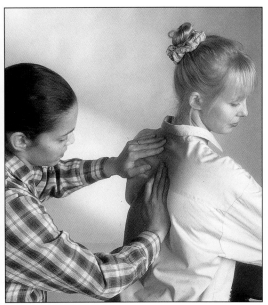

7 Allow the fingers to sink into the muscles around the shoulder blade. Repeat on the other side.

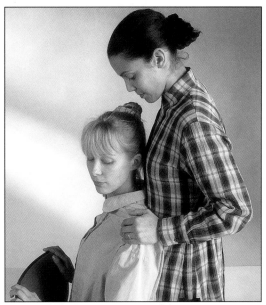

8 Place your hands on your partner's shoulder joints and press back towards yourself. This movement will give a gentle stretch to the upper chest.

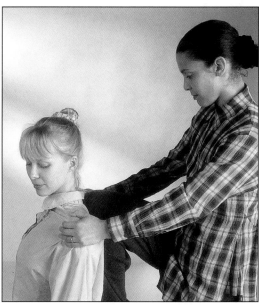

9 With care and balance, you can do this stretch with your leg pressing into your colleague's back.

HEALING MASSAGE

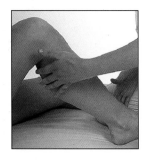

Massage can evoke many beneficial changes within the body, mind and spirit of the whole person. As well as relaxing stiff and aching muscles, it is a powerful treatment precisely because it works on both physical and psychological levels, and because it is able both to relax and invigorate the person receiving it. As the vicious circle of tension between mind and body is broken down by massage, the specific symptoms to which the tension gives rise can be alleviated.

To touch, caress and hold is a natural response to emotional or physical pain, and it is a practice found in every culture. During a massage, soft, flowing strokes calm and soothe the nervous system, stimulate the nerve-endings in the skin, and warm and loosen the superficial tissues. Deeper strokes remove tension from muscles and increase suppleness and mobility. Blood and lymph circulation is boosted, so that vital nutrients reach all the cells and toxins are eliminated. Revitalizing strokes invigorate energy levels and leave the skin with a healthy glow. Breathing deepens as the person becomes more relaxed and energized, increasing the intake of oxygen into the body and the expulsion of carbon dioxide from the lungs. Calm, still holds will enable the person to relax deeply and discharge pent-up feelings of stress.

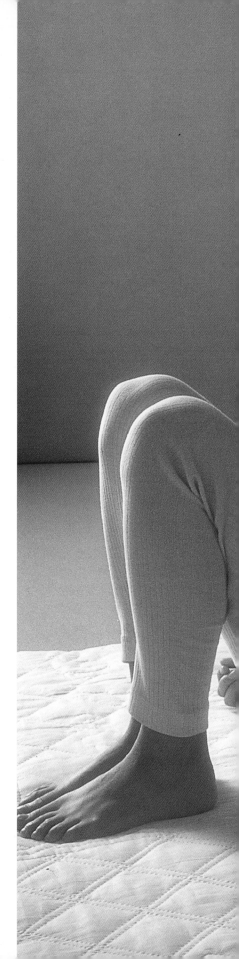

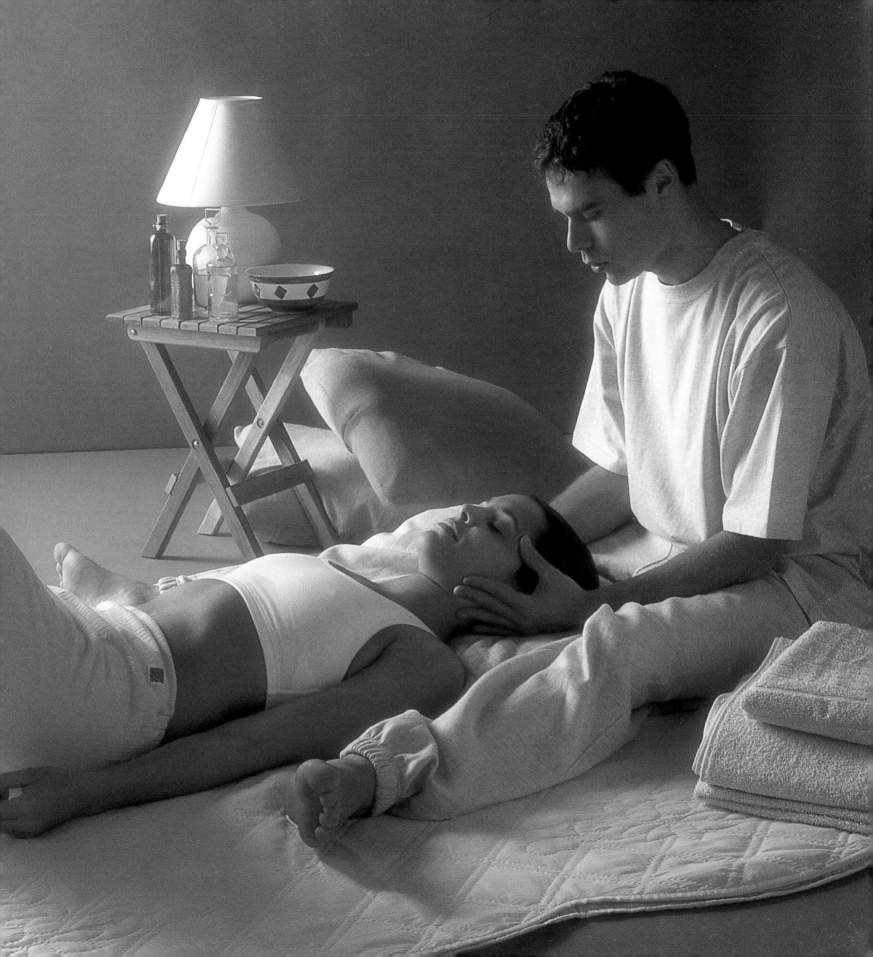

HEADACHE AND TENSION RELIEVER

One of the most common symptoms people experience when they are under stress is a tension headache; for some, this can become almost a daily pattern and may lead to migraine attacks. Any treatment should be given at the earliest stage, and massage is no exception. Just a few minutes of these soothing strokes may prevent major muscle spasm and pain.

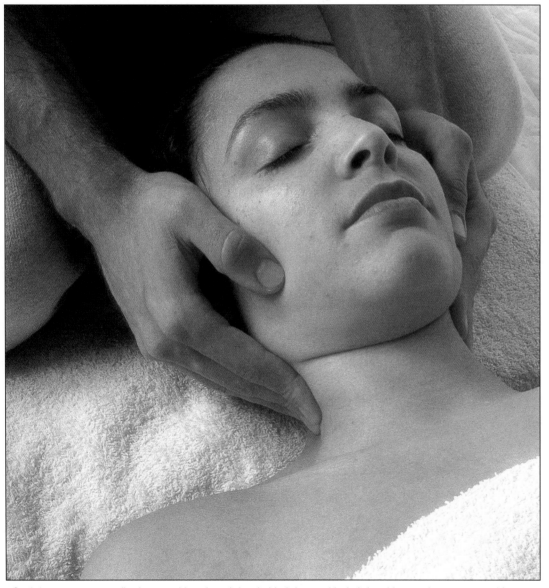

1 Ask your partner to lie down and kneel or sit just behind them, with their head in your lap or on a cushion.

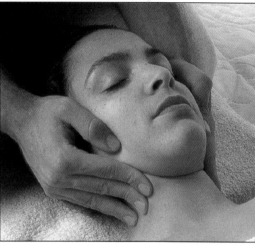

2 Using your fingertips, work with alternating circular friction strokes on the muscles on either side of your partner's neck.

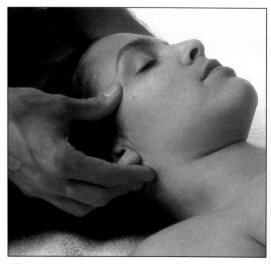

3 Continue circling, this time with both hands working at the same time, around the side of the head and behind the ears.

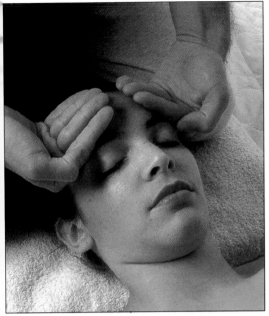

4 Smooth tension away from the temples with the backs or sides of your hands, using some gentle effleurage strokes.

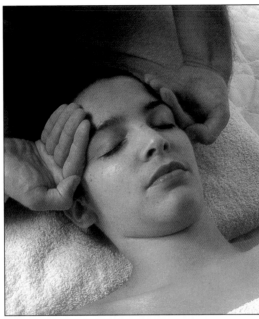

5 Gently draw the hands outwards across the forehead to soothe away worry lines.

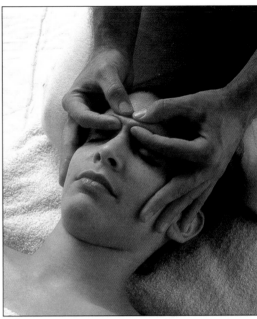

6 Pinch and squeeze along the line of the eyebrows, picking up the flesh between finger and thumb. Reduce the pressure as you work outward.

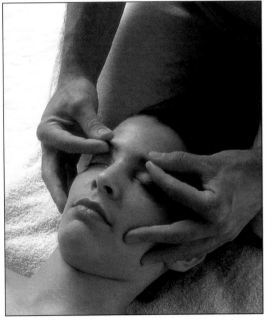

7 These muscles may be quite tender, so check with your partner and do not apply more pressure than is comfortable.

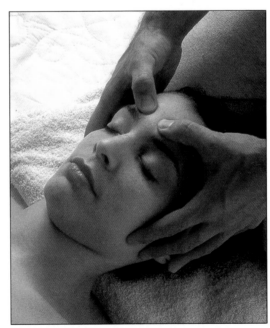

8 With your thumbs, use steady but firm pressure on the forehead, working outwards from between the eyebrows.

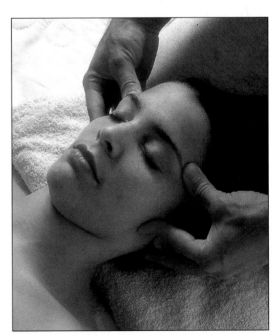

9 Work across the brow to the hairline using your thumbs. This covers many acupressure points and will release blocked energy.

SLEEP-ENHANCING FACIAL SOOTHER

If your partner has frequent problems with sleeping, or simply carries a lot of tension around in the facial muscles, this soothing programme may help. Apart from acting as an aid to relaxation, working on these muscles will smooth out worry lines and re-invigorate the face.

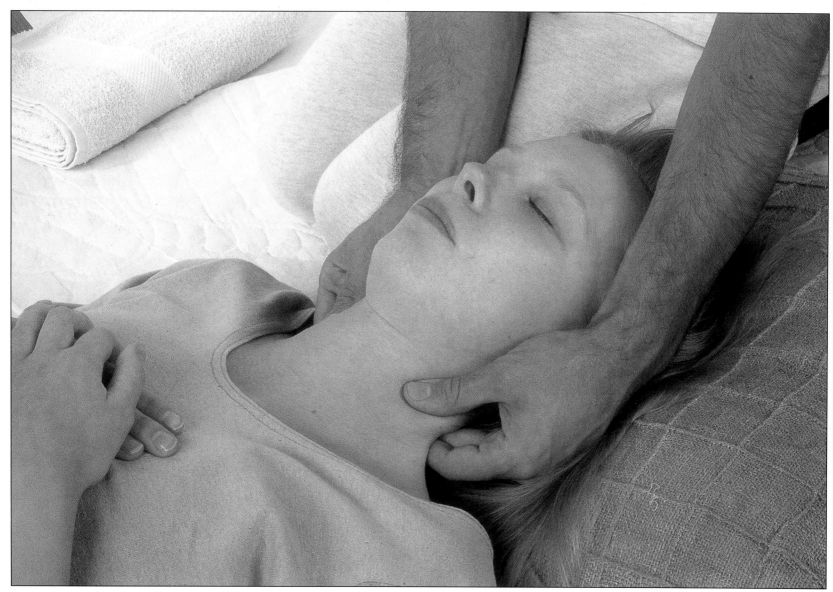

1 Kneeling behind your partner's head, with their head resting comfortably on a cushion, place both your hands under the neck. Pull very gently on the neck muscles, creating a little traction to stretch out the neck and head.

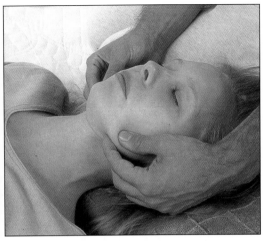

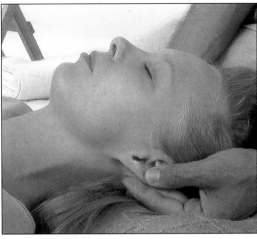

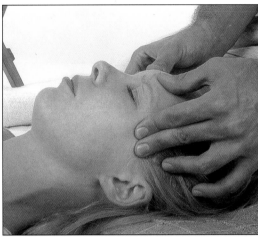

2 With your fingertips, make small circling friction movements along the jawline and over the cheeks. Use firm pressure but, as with all massage, avoid causing any discomfort. Try to work symmetrically, using both hands at the same time.

3 Pull gently with the fingertips and stretch the ears, working around from the earlobes to the top of the ears and back again.

4 Apply circling friction movements with your fingers or thumbs on the temples and forehead, lightening your touch as you work up the temples.

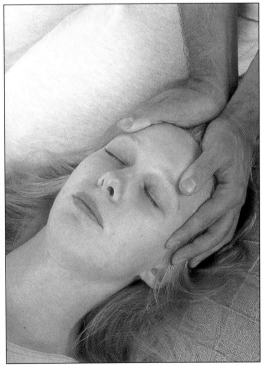

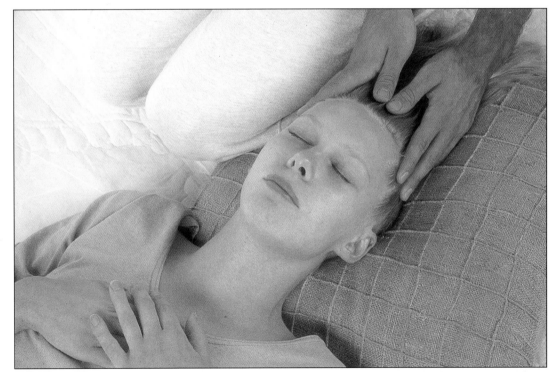

5 With the palms of your hands, smooth across the forehead, soothing the area you have worked on and easing out tension and worry lines.

6 Continue this movement, but now working your hands towards you, and extend it by stroking up into the hair to complete the sequence.

POOR CIRCULATION

Poor circulation to the extremities is quite common in cooler climates, and particularly in elderly people or those who do very little exercise. It can lead to more serious conditions, such as phlebitis or thrombosis, so it should not be neglected. Cold hands and feet can be warmed up initially by rubbing them briskly between your hands: the friction both warms the skin and stimulates the blood supply.

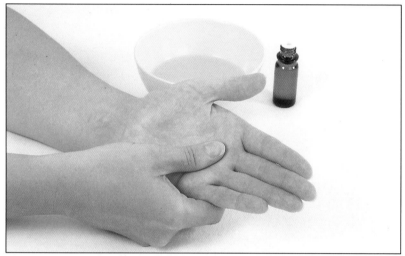

1 Using a little oil, massage the palm of the hand with a steady circular movement of the thumb.

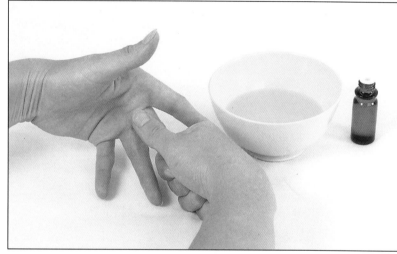

2 Squeeze down each of the fingers to stretch and loosen the joints, pushing towards the palm. Repeat steps 1 and 2 several times.

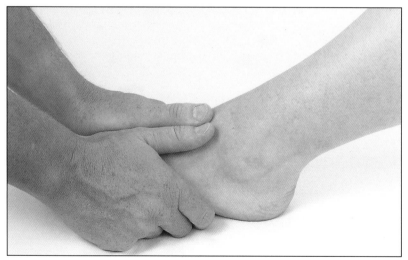

3 To stretch the foot, place both hands with the thumbs on top and fingers underneath, keeping a firm grip.

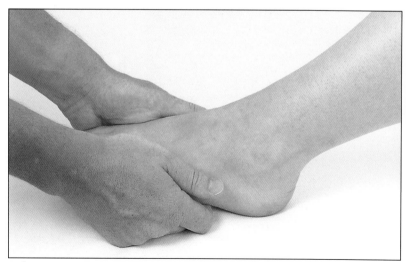

4 Move the thumbs outward, as if breaking a piece of bread. Repeat the movement several times, keeping the fingers still while moving your thumbs.

FLUID RETENTION

Excess fluid in the tissues, or oedema, can have a variety of causes. Fluid retention in the thighs and hips in women is often associated with a build-up of toxins, as is cellulite. In hot weather most people find that fluid retention is aggravated. A general detoxifying programme of diet, exercise and massage will usually help.

Massage the legs and thighs to improve the local circulation and so bring more blood and oxygen to the muscles. Firm effleurage movements are particularly helpful, always done in a direction towards the heart.

Inadequate circulation to the muscles is also a cause of cramp, especially if it comes on with exercise or effort. It is probably most common in the calves, but the acute and painful contraction can occur in any large muscles. For frequent leg cramps, regular massage of the legs and thighs is recommended. Essential oils such as juniper, lavender, marjoram, rosemary or black pepper will help to dilate the local blood vessels and encourage increased blood flow. Night cramps are likely as a combination of reduced circulation, tiredness and stress, and the whole person needs to be treated to alleviate this painful symptom.

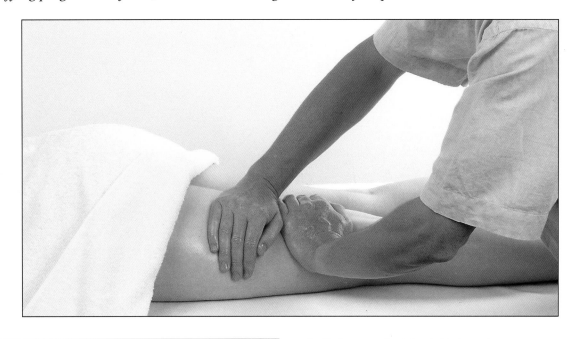

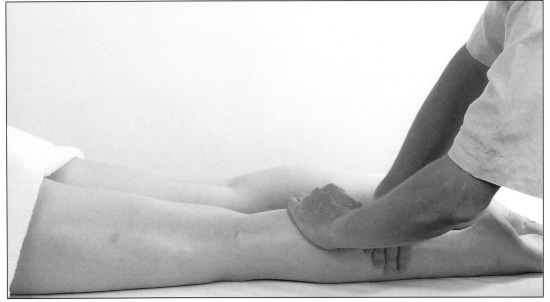

1 To improve circulation in the legs, place your hands on your partner's thigh and stroke upwards to the buttock several times using smooth effleurage movements. Keep the pressure light but steady, letting one hand follow the other.

2 Move your hands down to the calf and stroke up to the back of the knee a few times. Repeat these two steps, always starting the massage on the upper leg and always stroking towards the heart.

MASSAGE AND EXERCISE

Professional sportspeople value massage very highly. Used before exercise it helps to prepare the body for an increase in activity, not only by warming and loosening the muscles and joints – thereby helping to prevent cramp and injury – but also by stimulating the system physically and mentally. After an exercise session, massage speeds up the elimination of waste products, particularly lactic acid, by stimulating the lymphatic system. The accumulation of these toxins during exercise is the cause of much of the stiffness and pain that may otherwise be experienced afterwards.

STRAINS AND SPRAINS

A burning sensation under the skin is likely to indicate that muscles, fibres or ligaments have been strained – stretched beyond their natural limits. This is often the result of exercising without an adequate warm-up, or of over-exertion. A pre-exercise massage and warm-up routine will help prevent strains. Gently massaging the affected area will help speed recovery.

Sprains are more serious and are caused by violent wrenching of a joint, most commonly the ankle, wrist or knee. The surrounding muscles, ligaments and tendons may also be damaged and the affected area may be extremely painful and swollen. Apply an ice-pack or cold compress for 15–20 minutes to reduce the swelling. After this you can start to massage the area gently, taking care not to work directly on the swelling. Rest the joint as much as possible and use a support bandage.

A serious sprain should always be checked by a doctor in case a bone has been fractured, and a sprained knee always requires medical attention.

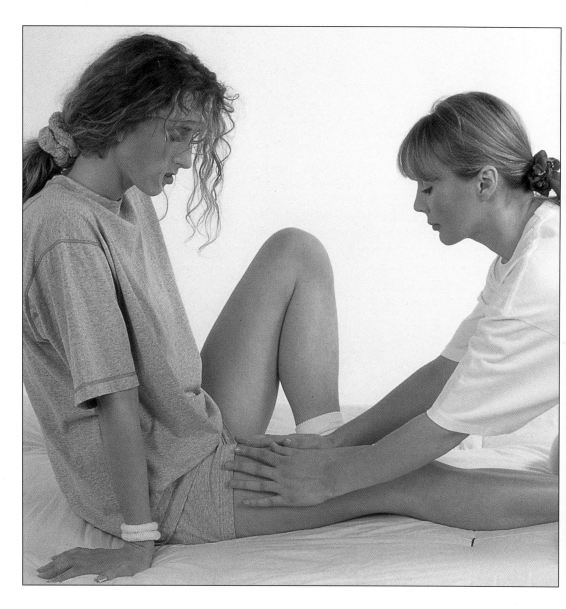

1 Avoid working directly on the swollen area (in this case the ankle). Start with gentle effleurage strokes working from the knee towards the thigh. Massaging in the direction of the lymph nodes in the groin will help drain away the fluids that have accumulated around the injured joint. Lightly stroke back to the knee. Repeat several times.

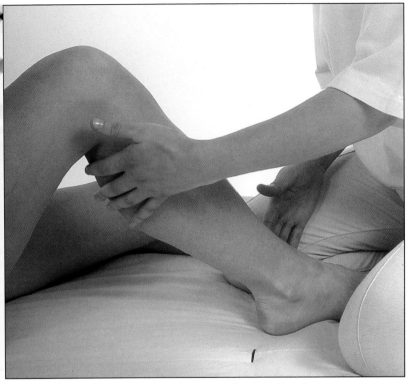

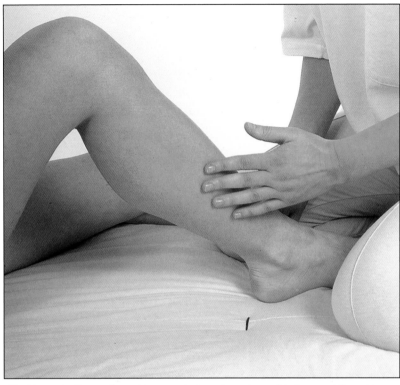

2 Help your partner to bend the affected leg. Continue the effleurage strokes on the lower leg, this time working from the ankle to the knee, alternating your hands. Repeat several times, then gently squeeze the calf with one hand, while the other supports the foot.

3 Concentrating on the ankle area, stroke extremely gently all around the ankle with short upward movements. Check that this is not causing discomfort.

ALLEVIATING BACKACHE

Back strain is the most common source of debilitating pain. Most sports put strain of some kind on the legs, buttocks and back, and previous injuries can make the back prone to recurrent pain. Falls and awkward landings are an inevitable part of many sports, but you should take care to avoid inappropriate or excessive exercise wherever possible. You should never subject your back to unnecessary strain. A regular and thorough back massage, particularly before exercise, can greatly reduce the likelihood of injury by loosening up the muscles and improving suppleness. Always consult a doctor, osteopath or chiropractor if you are in any doubt about the seriousness of a back problem.

ESSENTIAL OILS AND BLENDS FOR SPORT

Before exercise
For supple, toned muscles:
black pepper; ginger; rosemary; lavender; cypress; juniper; peppermint; grapefruit; orange.

To aid the respiratory system for aerobics:
eucalyptus; peppermint and rosemary; geranium.

For mental preparation before an event:
rosemary; lemon; lavender and chamomile.

To improve circulation:
rose and palmarosa.

After exercise
To soothe and prevent aching muscles:
eucalyptus; ginger and peppermint.

To eliminate stress following a competition:
lemon; nutmeg; clary sage; orange.

ALLEVIATING CRAMP

It is usually underused or ill-prepared muscles that go into cramp during exercise. Frequent cramps may indicate poor circulation or a deficiency of calcium or salt. Massage will improve circulation and alleviate the pain.

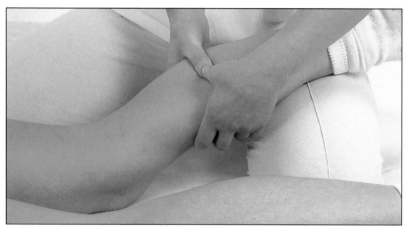

1 To relieve calf cramp, have your partner lie face down with the foot of the affected leg supported on your leg or a small pillow. Gradually apply direct thumb pressure into the centre of the cramped calf muscle for 8–10 seconds.

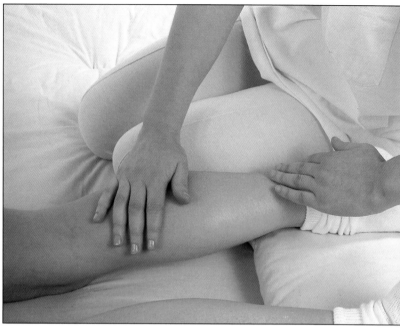

2 Do some effleurage strokes, working from ankle to thigh and back down again.

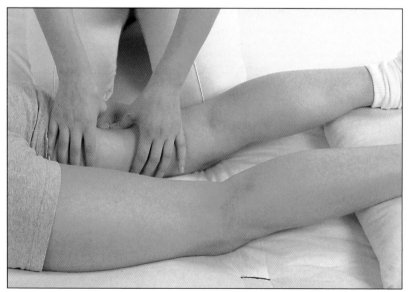

3 For hamstring cramp, raise the ankle on a small pillow and begin by massaging up the back of the thigh using alternate hands in slow, rhythmical stroking movements. Then apply static pressure to the middle of the thigh with the thumbs, holding for 8–10 seconds.

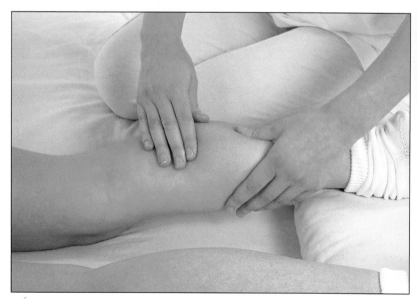

4 Firmly knead the calf muscle. Squeeze, press and release the muscle using one hand after the other. Finally, do some soothing effleurage strokes up from ankle to thigh and back down again.

SELF-HELP CRAMP STRETCHES

Cramp is a sudden and involuntary contraction of a muscle, and you can help to alleviate the pain by stretching the muscle gently to help it relax.

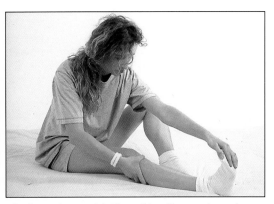

1 A good way of dealing with calf cramp is to sit down with the affected leg straight and stretch the toes towards you. Hold this position for 8 seconds, then release. Repeat a few times, until the spasm seems to be lessening, then knead your calf muscle using firm pressure. When the muscle feels relaxed, switch to effleurage strokes, working up the leg.

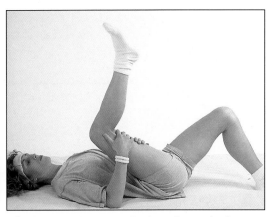

2 For hamstring cramp, lie down flat on the floor, with the affected leg raised and the other knee bent. Stretch the muscle by pulling the thigh gently towards the chest. Firmly stroke up the back of your thigh for 8–10 seconds. Start to knead the back of the thigh until you feel the muscles begin to relax. Finally, stroke over the area to soothe it.

TENNIS ELBOW

Pain on the outside of the elbow may be due to inflammation of the tendon resulting from overuse. It may be caused by sporting activities, but can also result from digging in the garden or lifting heavy objects. Avoid repeating the activity for a week or two to allow the inflammation to subside.

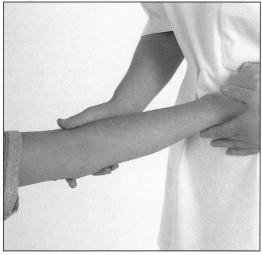

1 Support your partner's wrist in one hand and use soothing effleurage strokes along both sides of the arm, stroking from the wrist to the elbow and back again. Repeat several times.

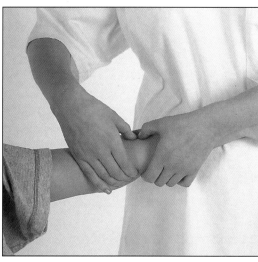

2 Rest your partner's hand against your side. Continue to work up their arm, from the wrist to the elbow and back, making small circular movements with both thumbs, paying particular attention to the muscles in the forearm.

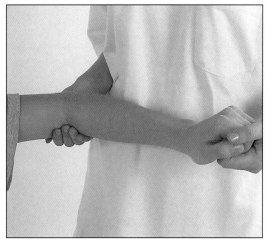

3 Secure your partner's hand in yours, and with your other hand supporting their elbow, flex your partner's elbow forward.

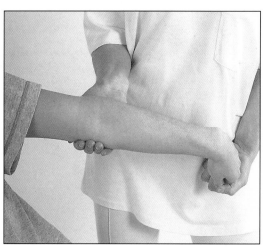

4 Bring the hand back, to give the tendons that are attached to the bones a good stretch.

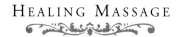

SENSUAL MASSAGE

As well as releasing stresses and tensions from the muscles, massage is a wonderful way to enhance a relationship by increasing caring, sharing touch. If your relationship seems to have got into a rut and sexual energy is low, you can revitalize yourselves with some soothing massage strokes.

The skin is so highly sensitive that it is able to transmit and receive loving messages and feelings conveyed through the hands, nourishing not only the body but the mind and emotions. Massage can become a means of deep communication, a way to show how much you care for each other.

It is important to take a little extra time to create the right environment so as to make the whole experience a real treat – time for you both in a hurried world. Make the room extra warm and wear minimal clothing or undress fully, covering your partner with warm towels if necessary. You may want to play some of your favourite soothing music. Arrange soft lighting or, better still, work by candlelight.

Gentle effleurage strokes should be the mainstay of a sensual massage. Use a little more oil than usual to help the strokes flow more easily.

Intuition will play a large part in your massage, as you discover which areas have the strongest impact on your partner's senses. It isn't just the most obvious erogenous zones that bring pleasure: pay attention to the back of the neck, scalp, solar plexus, the inside of the elbows, and the hands and feet, to make the massage a highly pleasurable and sensual experience for both of you.

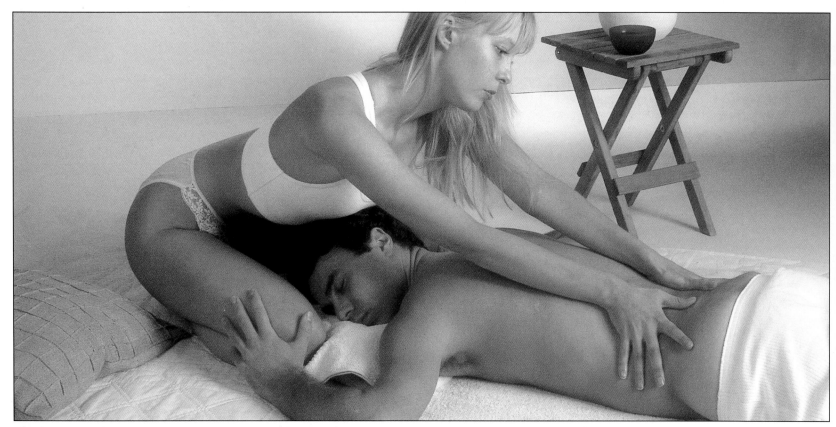

1 Using gentle effleurage strokes, place your hands on either side of the spine and glide right down the back from the shoulders. Move your hands out to the side and up the back again. Repeat several times, making your hands soft and pliable so that they mould and encompass the shapes and curves of your partner's body.

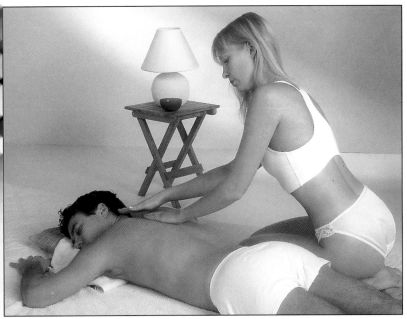

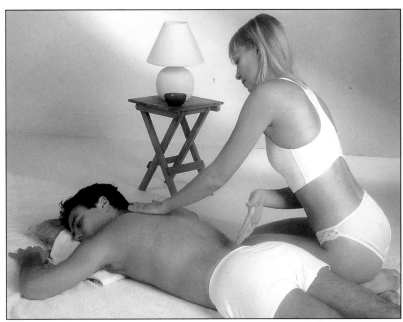

2 Kneeling beside your partner's hips, stroke down the centre of the back with one hand following the other smoothly, as if you were stroking a cat.

3 As one hand lifts off at the lower back, start again with the other hand at the neck in soothing, languid strokes.

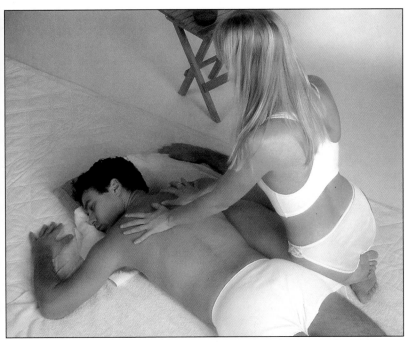

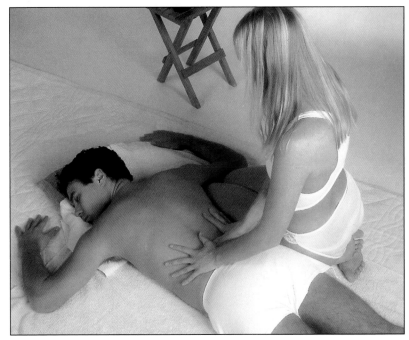

4 Place both of your hands on your partner's upper back and stroke outwards in a fan shape. Shape your hands to the sides of the body, then draw them down before sliding them lightly around and back to the centre of the back.

5 Work down the back, including the buttocks, repeating the fanning action.

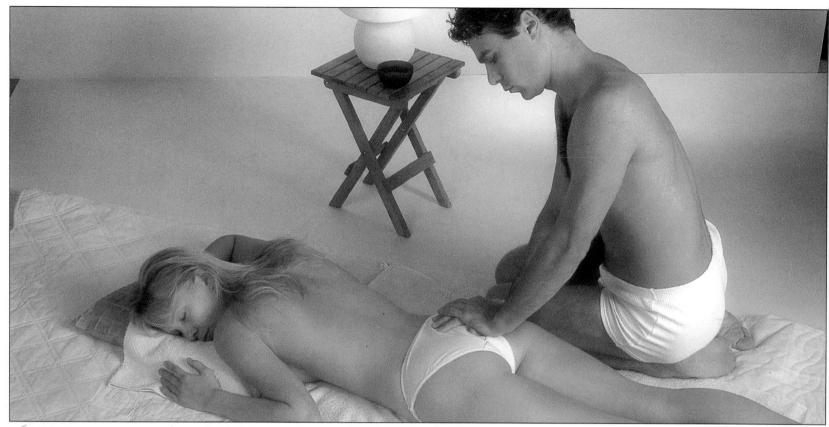

6 Use a firm, steady circling action on the buttocks. These are large, powerful muscles that may be able to take quite firm pressure if your partner desires it, but avoid giving any discomfort.

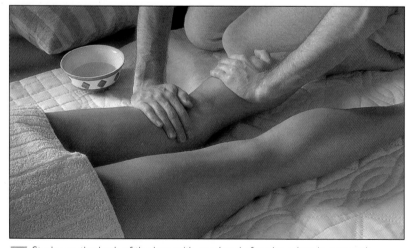

7 Stroke up the back of the legs, with one hand after the other, in a smooth, flowing motion.

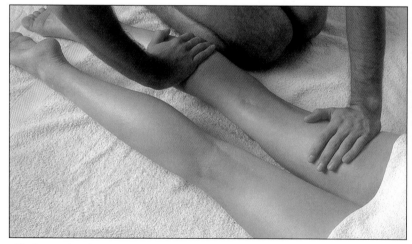

8 As one hand reaches the buttocks, start on the calf with the other hand, keeping a steady rhythm. This overlapping stroke creates the sensation of many hands caressing the body, and feels particularly wonderful on the legs and arms.

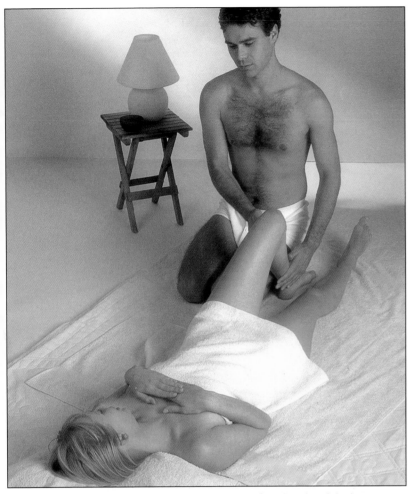

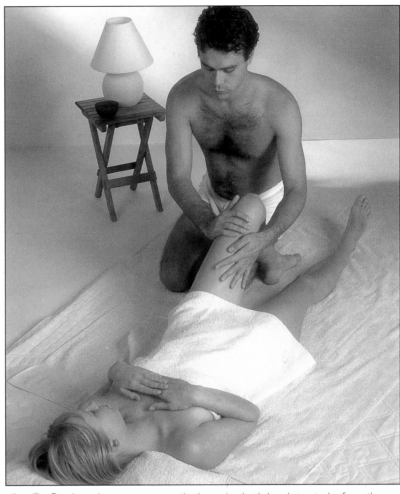

9 Turn your partner over and stroke up the front of the legs; bend the knee to help the muscles relax completely.

10 Continue the movement up the leg, using both hands to stroke from the knees up to the thighs.

11 Effleurage may also be used on the front of the body, kneeling behind your partner's head. Be careful not to press in with your thumbs. All these movements should make for a truly sensual experience, and help put your partner back in touch with their body – and maybe yours too.

SENSUAL OILS

When choosing essential oils for sensual massage, the most important consideration is personal taste. The massage will not be a pleasurable experience if either of you finds the blend of aromas disagreeable. Allow an intuitive choice to guide you in making a blend of aromas that you both find appealing.

There are, however, a few oils that seem to have a universal appeal: jasmine, rose, rosewood, sandalwood and ylang ylang. These oils are the embodiment of luxury and are indeed some of the most precious. They have a warming and enveloping quality, freeing the mind and opening it to the exotic and romantic. To add spice and stimulation to your chosen blend, add either black pepper or frankincense.

ENHANCING YOUR MASSAGE

Once you have achieved a good grounding in the basic techniques of massage, you can further enhance your skills by using a massage couch, and by experimenting with the use of additional pillows.

WORKING AT A COUCH

While some people prefer to kneel and give a massage at floor level, working at a couch increases your mobility, as you can move more freely when on your feet. This puts less stress on your posture, enabling you to bring length to your spine and neck and a relaxed width to your shoulders. As with the kneeling position, your movement should come from the lower half of your body to avoid strain on your back.

There are many different types of massage couch to choose from, designed for various styles of massage and in a wide price range. It is important to choose a couch built to the correct height for you: if you stand with your fists loosely clenched and let your arms hang down by your sides, you should be able to rest your knuckles comfortably on the surface of the couch. The width of a massage couch should be a minimum of 65–80cm/26–32in, in order to support the whole body securely and allow sufficient space for the arms to relax on the couch. The length is normally a minimum of 180cm/72in. Foam padding, covered with vinyl, should be firm but comfortable.

A face cradle can be added to the table, or a face hole cut into its surface, to enable the head and neck to be supported straight. Some people find it difficult to lie in a prone position as it necessitates an awkward angle of the neck.

If you are planning to set up a mobile massage practice and want a portable, folding couch, it is important to choose one that is easy to carry. You will need to find the right balance between stability, strength and ease of transportation.

USING PILLOWS AND TOWELS TO EASE TENSION

Postural tension remains in the body even when your partner is lying down on the couch to receive a massage. A prolonged period of resting on a flat surface can even exacerbate physical strain, especially in the major joints of the body. The more you massage, the more you will be able to see where someone is holding tension. For example, an individual may have a particularly swayed lower back, indicating stress in the pelvic region, or the neck may be contracted or sore, making it extremely difficult to lie comfortably. Using pillows or rolled towels to support key areas of the body can ease the structural tension, enabling your partner to relax and enjoy the highly beneficial experience of massage to the full.

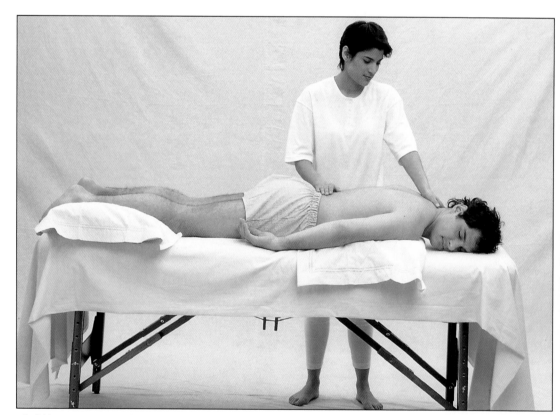

1 When your partner is lying in a prone position, place one pillow just below the knees. The benefit of taking the strain out of these joints will further relax the pelvis and lower back. A pillow under the front of the chest will allow the shoulders to fall forwards, opening up the upper back and creating space between the shoulder blades. The added support will also help to lengthen and relax the back.

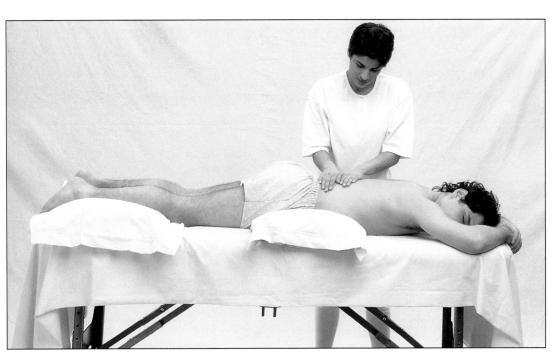

2 Pain in the lower back may be caused by an excessive curve in the base of the spine, or a chronic pattern of tension in the pelvic region. A pillow placed supportively under the abdomen can redress the postural imbalance during the massage, helping the lumbar region to relax under your touch.

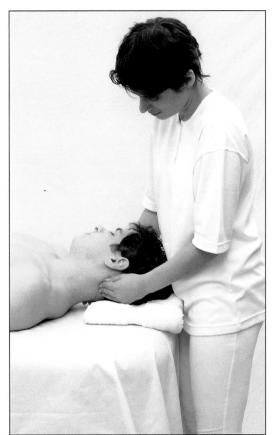

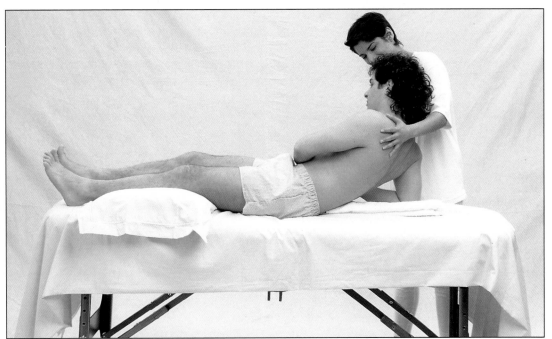

3 Tension in the chest and ribcage can cause muscles to contract, pulling the shoulders forwards so that they are unable to rest on the table during massage. Ease this uncomfortable posture by placing a towel, folded into a thin strip, under and along the length of the spine. This will enable the chest to expand and the shoulders to fall back. Help your partner into the supine position so that the towel remains in the correct place.

4 Constriction in the muscle attachments at the base of the skull will shorten the neck muscles, causing the head to contract backwards. Bring a sense of length and relief to this area by placing a thin, folded towel under the ridge of the skull to lift the head slightly upwards and to extend the neck.

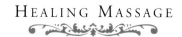

BODY ENERGY AND AURIC MASSAGE

Knowledge of the body's auric and energy vibrations has always existed in spiritual and healing practices, but has been largely ignored by modern medicine and science. The influence of this subtle energy field on our health and well-being can be explored through massage, which can bring to the aura the benefits of healing and balance, helping to protect the physical body from ill-health and emotional disturbance.

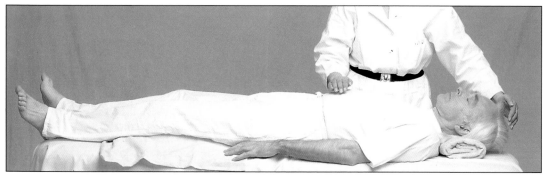

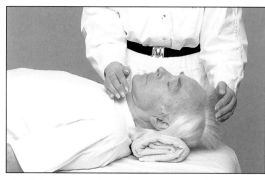

1 Make sure your partner is lying down comfortably and feeling warm and safe. Take time to become still and meditative within yourself by focusing your attention on your own body and breathing. This will help your hands tune into subtle energy vibrations. Begin with a session of healing holds to bring a sense of unity to the body and restore equilibrium to the mind.

2 Raise your hands to shoulder level and let them drift down with sensitivity, to feel the edge of the aura as a tangible but subtle vibration. Enter this energy field, resting your hands, without weight, on your partner's body. Tune into your partner's essential energy, and hold until intuition tells you to move your hands.

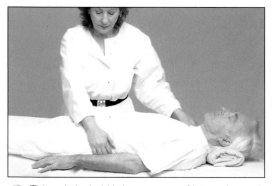

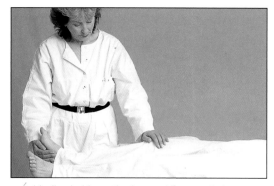

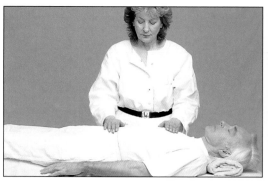

3 This polarity hold brings a sense of integration and balance to both sides of the body. When at your partner's left side, place your left hand on the right shoulder and your right hand on the left hip. Imagine a current of energy passing between your hands.

4 Healing holds on the legs and feet can help to earth the physical body and stabilize the emotions. Start with a hip and foot hold to connect the whole leg. Then place your right hand over the knee, keeping your left hand on the hip. Finally, place your left hand over the knee while cupping your right hand beneath the sole of the foot.

5 When your partner is calm, massage the aura in smooth, slow, rhythmic strokes towards the feet, working down the body and over the limbs one at a time. Do this three times: start by clearing the spiritual plane (45–60cm/18–24in above the body), then move to the emotional plane (15–20cm/6–8in) and finally, to the physical level (5–7.5cm/2–3in). To finish, let your hands hover over your partner's abdomen and heart, before settling gently on the body.

USEFUL ADDRESSES

ORGANIZATIONS

Association of Physical and Natural Therapists
93 Parkhurst Road
Horley, Surrey
UK RH6 8EX
Tel: 01293 775467

Institute for Complementary Medicine
Unit 4, Tavern Quay
London
UK SE16 1QZ
Tel: 0171 237 5165

New York Institute of Massage
PO Box 645
Buffalo
NY 14231
USA
Tel: 800 884 NYIM

PRACTITIONERS AND COURSES

Champneys
Chesham Road
Wiggington
Tring
Hertfordshire
UK HP23 6HY
Tel: 01442 863351

Grayshott Hall
Headley Road
Grayshott
Nr Hindhead
Surrey
UK GU26 6JJ
Tel: 01428 604331

Henlow Grange
Henlow
Bedfordshire
UK SG16 6BD
Tel: 01462 811111

London College of Massage
5 Newman Passage
London
UK W1P 3PF
Tel: 0171 323 3574

London School of Sports Massage
88 Cambridge Street
London
UK SW1V 4QG
Tel: 0171 233 5962

Massage Training Institute
24 Highbury Grove
London
UK N5 2EA
Tel: 0171 226 5313

American Massage Therapy Association
820 Davies Street
Evanston
IL 60201
USA

Boulder School of Massage Therapy
PO Box 4573
Boulder
CO 80306
USA

The Connecticut Center for Massage Therapy
75 Kitts Lane
Newington
CT 06111
USA

Australian Natural Therapists Association
PO Box 522
Sutherland
NSW 2232
Australia

South African Institute of Health and
Beauty Therapists
PO Box 56318
Pinegowrie
22123
Johannesburg
South Africa

FURTHER READING

el Dawes and Fiona Harrold, *Massage Cures*,
Thorsons, 1990
orge Downing, *The Massage Book*, Wildwood
House, 1973
iona Harrold, *The Massage Manual*, Headline,
1992
Nitya Lacroix, *Massage for Total Relaxation*,
Dorling Kindersley, 1991

—*Sensual Massage*, Dorling Kindersley, 1989
Lucinda Lidell, *The Massage Book*, Ebury Press,
1984
Clare Maxwell-Hudson, *The Complete Book of
Massage*, Dorling Kindersley, 1988
Sara Thomas, *Massage for Common Ailments*,
Sidgwick & Jackson, 1989
Jacqueline Young, *Self Massage*, Thorsons, 1992

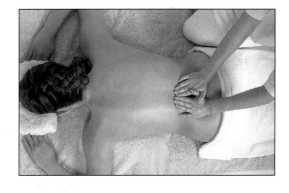

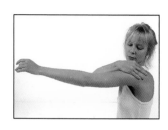
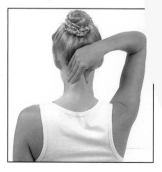